Kim —
Happy 40th
Birthday!
Enjoy your special
day! Hugs —
Auntie Mar 2020

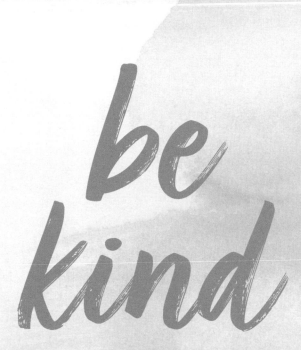

be kind

A YEAR OF KINDNESS,
ONE WEEK AT A TIME

MELISSA BURMESTER & JACLYN LINDSEY
founders of kindess.org

ROCK
POINT

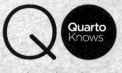

Inspiring | Educating | Creating | Entertaining

Brimming with creative inspiration, how-to projects, and useful information to enrich your everyday life, Quarto Knows is a favorite destination for those pursuing their interests and passions. Visit our site and dig deeper with our books into your area of interest: Quarto Creates, Quarto Cooks, Quarto Homes, Quarto Lives, Quarto Drives, Quarto Explores, Quarto Gifts, or Quarto Kids.

First published in 2020 by Rock Point, an imprint of The Quarto Group,
142 West 36th Street, 4th Floor, New York, NY 10018, USA
T (212) 779-4972 F (212) 779-6058 www.QuartoKnows.com

Rock Point titles are also available at discount for retail, wholesale, promotional and bulk purchase. For details, contact the Special Sales Manager by email at specialsales@quarto.com or by mail at The Quarto Group, Attn: Special Sales Manager, 100 Cummings Center Suite, 265D, Beverly, MA 01915, USA.

10 9 8 7 6 5 4 3 2

ISBN: 978-1-63106-684-9

Library of Congress Control Number: 2019956366

Publisher: Rage Kindelsperger
Creative Director: Laura Drew
Managing Editor: Cara Donaldson
Senior Editor: Erin Canning
Cover and Interior Design: Merideth Harte

Printed in China CC072020

To Abel and Amelia,
for motivating us to build
the kind of world we
want you to grow up in.

CONTENTS

FOREWORD: The Science of Kindness 8

INTRODUCTION: 10

HOW TO USE THIS BOOK: 14

52 Weeks of Kindness

WEEK 1: Q & A with Eli 19

WEEK 2: 1,000 Kilometers of Kindness 23

WEEK 3: The Gift of Gratitude 27

WEEK 4: I've Got Your Back 31

WEEK 5: There Is Kindness in Clarity 35

WEEK 6: Q & A with Carlos Navarro 39

WEEK 7: The Lasting Warmth of a Simple Gesture 43

WEEK 8: Appreciating a Stranger's Generosity 47

WEEK 9: A Lifetime of Kindness 51

WEEK 10: Q & A with Eric Hutcherson 55

WEEK 11: Reconnecting with Mother Nature 59

WEEK 12: The "F" Word 63

WEEK 13: You Are Not Alone 67

WEEK 14: Kindness across Difference 71

WEEK 15: Mentoring with Thoughtfulness 75

WEEK 16: A Welcome like No Other   79

WEEK 17: An Impactful Umbrella   83

WEEK 18: Q & A with Amy Jo Martin   87

WEEK 19: A Gift, Not Judgment, for the Mom of a Special Needs Child   91

WEEK 20: To Spend, to Save, or to Give?   95

WEEK 21: Friendship and Inclusion   99

WEEK 22: The Power of a Power Nap   103

WEEK 23: A Letter to the Love of My Life, My Kind, Beautiful, and Inspiring Wife, Hellie   107

WEEK 24: Q & A with Sebastian Terry   111

WEEK 25: Bonded over Kidneys   115

WEEK 26: Giving the Gift of Time and Knowledge   119

WEEK 27: Are You Smiling at Me?   123

WEEK 28: A Restaurant That Served Dignity   127

WEEK 29: One Small Act Changed the Course of My Life   131

WEEK 30: Q & A with Michelle Garside   135

WEEK 31: The Care Package   139

WEEK 32: Forgiveness May Take Time   143

WEEK 33: The Day You Saved My Life   147

WEEK 34: Thoughts from an Almost Centenarian   151

WEEK 35: The Lazy Litterer   155

WEEK 36: Kindness Is a Universal Language   159

WEEK 37: From Neighbors to Friends   163

WEEK 38: A Letter to Myself   167

WEEK 39: Quiet Kindness   171

WEEK 40: Q & A with Dr. Megan Jones Bell   175

WEEK 41: Finding Grace When Someone Is Unkind   179

WEEK42: Kindness Is a Muscle   183

WEEK 43: Getting Empathy from an Unexpected Source   187

WEEK 44: Giving Credit Where Credit Is Due   191

WEEK 45: Kinder.   195

WEEK 46: Q & A with Tom Tait   199

WEEK 47: Have I Ever Thanked You?   203

WEEK 48: Taking the Fear out of Giving Blood   207

WEEK 49: Q & A with Henry Hitchcox   211

WEEK 50: Collective Kindness Saves the Day   215

WEEK 51: Q & A with Eric Ripert   219

WEEK 52: Dear You   223

NOTES   227

KIND ACTS CHECKLIST   230

BIBLIOGRAPHY   232

ACKNOWLEDGMENTS   236

ABOUT THE AUTHORS   238

ABOUT KINDNESS.ORG   240

"Together, our ripples of kindness can create massive waves of change."

—KINDNESS.ORG

Foreword > THE SCIENCE OF KINDNESS

What is kindness? Why are people kind? What are the different types of kindness? How does kindness contribute to a happy and fulfilling life? And how can we make the world a kinder place?

In recent years, science has made immense progress in answering these questions—and our goal at Kindlab, the research hub for kindness.org, is to take the science further still.

Humans are kind because we are an intensely social species. We have lived in social groups for the past fifty million years, and throughout this time we have relied on cooperative relationships with others in order to survive and thrive. Kindness is a way of kick-starting and maintaining these relationships. Thus, we can explain why people are kind to their families, friends, spouses, community members, and even strangers. We can explain why kindness comes in many forms—including love, loyalty, camaraderie, compassion, reciprocity, respect, generosity, gratitude, fairness, forgiveness, heroism, and humility. We can explain why we find investing in these relationships rewarding, and why helping others makes us happy. And we can explain why most people are kind most of the time.

Most people, most of the time, but not everyone, always. What stops people from being kinder? There are many reasons. For example, some people lack the *incentive*—they don't care or don't see the point. Some people lack *information*—they would like to help, but they don't know what to do, or worry about what might happen if they get it wrong. And some people feel *isolated*—they would like to help, but they don't want to act alone for fear their efforts will be wasted.

Kindlab uses the latest insights from the science of kindness—the biological underpinnings, the psychological circuitry, and the social conditions that foster it—to design more effective interventions and programs for cultivating kindness at scale. We help people overcome these obstacles and make it easier for them to choose kindness.

To provide additional **incentives**, we use techniques from experimental psychology to measure the costs and benefits of kindness, and to show how even apparently insignificant acts of kindness can have a big impact.

To provide the missing **information**, we curate ideas for how to be kind and subject them to rigorous real-world testing by our citizen scientists.

And to overcome the feeling of **isolation**, our online community creates the common knowledge needed to reassure people that they are not acting alone, that their efforts are not futile, that they are appreciated, and that by acting together, they can achieve more than acting alone.

So, enjoy the science and stories presented in *Be Kind*, and join us in making the world a kinder place!

—*Dr. Oliver Scott Curry*, RESEARCH DIRECTOR AT KINDNESS.ORG

Introduction

We never dreamed this is what we'd be doing when we grew up, yet, it's clear in retrospect that this is always where both our paths would lead.

JACLYN

I tell people I'm a Florida girl. Even though Brooklyn has been my home for eight years, my heart belongs to the beach. It's where I feel most whole. It's where I was raised, part of a big, beautifully blended family that includes seven full, half-, and step-siblings. My brothers, sisters, and I learned about the power of generosity from our parents at an early age. Like many childhoods, there were good days and bad, but I most cling to the memories that give me what feels like a DNA-deep passion for helping people.

A few years ago, while at a crossroads of life and career, struggling with what to do next, I went to where I feel most comfortable and sat on a beach. I listened to the waves of wisdom and prayerfully asked what my personal mission was—what difference could I make each day? "Inspire Kindness and Generosity" is what materialized onto the pages of my journal. It was not exactly the clarity I was looking for, and yet, it was the most obvious answer I could have been given. Having grappled with bullying, self-esteem issues, and drug abuse, and ultimately finding a belief system that saved me, I had been filled with a deep conviction that at our core, kindness was something that could connect us all. I wanted more of it for myself, and I wanted it for the world. I wanted it because it felt like the clearest language of my personal faith that I could fully understand and speak to others.

Little did I know, and I'd soon discover, that this was a word that was bubbling to the top for so many people around me. There was one person who would soon become more than just a friend and colleague I saw every so often, but my co-founder on this journey.

MELISSA

I tell people that I am still a work in progress. Hah! When I landed on the focus of kindness, I was coming out of a season of self-reflection and facing the realization that I needed to make some changes in my life.

My mom says she worried about me when I was little because I was "too sweet"—if there weren't enough chairs at a table, I was the one without one. And then one day when I was in first grade, she found me after school, hands on hips, standing protectively in front of a neighborhood girl who was being bullied by a group of older kids. "I don't care what you say about her, she is my friend!" I declared. My mom was a little less worried after that—she saw my strength. Kindness no matter the personal cost, I do think that's who I was as a kid. But as I grew older and moved through my career, I lost that part of myself.

I became the typical busy New Yorker who didn't talk to my neighbors or make eye contact in the streets. I was prioritizing results over people at work, and work over friends. I didn't answer the phone enough when my family called. The empathy was still there, but I wasn't making the time to act on it.

Years later, I was burnt-out. My dad's health was in decline, and I felt like there were decisions and daily micro-actions that I was getting wrong. Something had to change. After a lot of thought, I had a direction (that I had yet to say out loud to anyone): I was ready to leave my job and no matter what I did next, I wanted to focus on being kind. Coincidentally, Jaclyn was the first person I told. I prefaced it with "don't laugh at me" because I thought the idea was irrational, having no notion that she had already landed in the same direction.

To be honest, we occasionally get it wrong. It's easy to feel inadequate while leading an organization focused on kindness. But we are committed to keeping at it—research, practice, mistakes, kind redos, continuous improvement. Kindness is a choice. Learning how to choose kindness more often—both when it is easy and when it is hard—is now a life mission. If everyone was just 10 percent kinder, how different would our world be?

Our goal for this book is that it will push you just a little bit outside your comfort zone and help you flex your kindness muscle. The scientific facts have all been vetted through Kindlab, the stories are all true (though some of the names have been changed), and the kind act suggestions have been evaluated for their cost and benefit ratio. Our hope is that by the end of the book you come to the same conclusion as us: every kind act matters.

Most importantly, we believe that we are all in this together, so we want to hear from you . . . we mean it! Tell us how the kind acts go, and share your ideas and suggestions. And thank you for choosing kindness.

—*Jaclyn & Melissa*

How to Use This Book

Be Kind takes the three elements of our mission, to **educate** and **inspire** people to **choose** kindness, and lays it out in a guide for you to experience a year of kindness, week by week.

Each of the fifty-two weeks includes a relevant research finding (learn), a reflection on the impact of kindness (reflect), and a kind act suggestion (do). There are also quotes from notable thinkers scattered throughout and a notes section in the back for jotting down thoughts, ideas, and more. We designed this book to be read one week at a time. Of course, no matter how you choose to experience this book, whether you read it cover to cover or dip in and out of it when the mood strikes you, we hope you use it as a reference and a reminder of all the good out in the world and how you can help contribute to it.

LEARN

Through our research arm, Kindlab, we've evaluated hundreds of academic papers related to kindness and conducted our own original research. For this book, we also invited a variety of scientists, researchers, and thought leaders to help us paint the picture of what kindness means in today's world. We start each week with a fact, statistic, or finding that we think is worth knowing.

REFLECT

Our research has found that even the smallest of kind acts can have a significant impact. These true stories, from people in our lives and the kindness.org community, demonstrate the power of kindness. They are shared as anecdotes, gratitude letters, and Q & As.

DO

The kind act suggestions have been evaluated and tested, but they are meant to be prompts that you should feel free to iterate upon. Some acts may feel easy, while others may push you outside your comfort zone. If you get to an act that you're unsure about or that you're already doing regularly, adapt it to what feels right for you.

Finally, we're here to support you! If you have a question or suggestion, reach out. Join us in building a database of Recommended Kind Acts and ultimately help build a kinder world. **You can visit kindness.org/bekind or email us at bekind@kindness.org.** We reply to every single message we receive, and can't wait to hear your story.

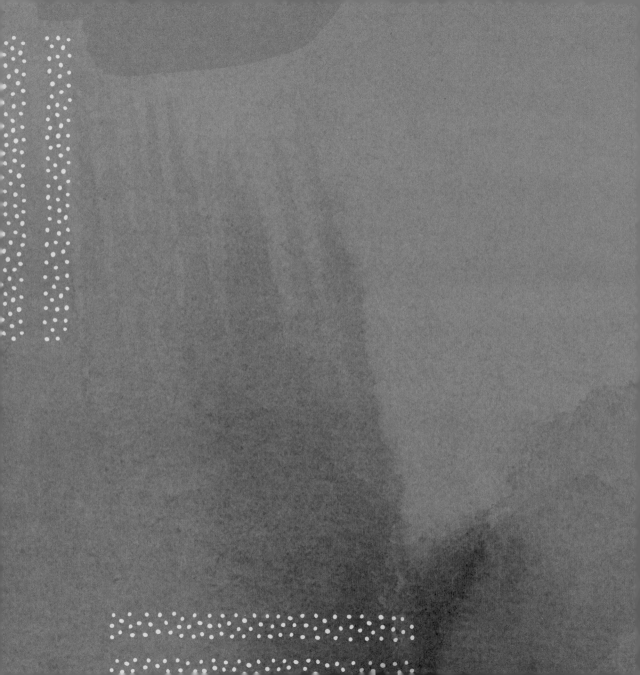

volunteer
say good morning
donate blood

say thank you
apologize

smile at a stranger
be nice online
encourage others

not fighting
friend

mentor someone

pick up litter
compliment someone

donate money

pay it forward

take someone to lunch

be supportive

bring snacks for co-workers
help someone in need
send a thank-you note

like social media posts

listen

hold the door

reconnect with an old
forgive someone

learn >

Let's start with the basics, the ABCs of kindness: **A**ction intended to **B**enefit the recipient, typically accompanied by an emotional **C**omponent.

(KINDNESS.ORG)

reflect ›

Q & A WITH ELI

Eli is seven years old.

Mom: *What does kindness mean to you?*

Eli: It means being nice to people and helping them when they need help.

Mom: *Tell me more . . .*

Eli: Well, like on the playground, if you see someone playing alone, you could invite them to play with you or go play with them.

Mom: *Are there times you've been kind at school?*

Eli: Someone dropped their Play-Doh on the floor. I picked it up for them.

Mom: *How did they react?*

Eli: They smiled and said thank you. That's another way to be kind, saying please and thank you.

Fast-forward to five minutes later . . .

Eli: And Mommy, it's very important to be kind to EVERYONE. NO MATTER WHAT! Because we're all unique. And that's a good thing.

do >

What does kindness mean to you?

Chances are, you've experienced kindness in many different ways at many different times, on both the giving and receiving ends. But in your own words, how do you define "kindness"? What actions come to mind? Take five minutes and write down what kindness means in your life.

learn >

Kindness is a meta-value that has the power to transform our world for the better. It encompasses acts of:

altruism

bravery compassion

decency empathy fairness

forgiveness friendship

generosity gratitude humility

love loyalty mercy munificence

trust respect sympathy

understanding

(KINDNESS.ORG)

reflect >

1,000 KILOMETERS OF KINDNESS

Ruth and her partner, Oli, spent 2018 cycling from Bristol, United Kingdom, to Bangkok, Thailand. They cycled over ten thousand kilometers and crossed twenty-two countries seeking recipes for kindness. Here is an excerpt from Ruth's personal reflections while on the road.

About midway through our journey, we had learned about the terrorist attack on a group of cyclists in Tajikistan and were fielding concerns from parents and friends overseas. Entering Tajikistan was a conflicting and confusing time. By then we had experienced kindness in the most profound ways. And we knew that one terrible experience didn't reflect the entire region. Oli's mum suggested flying over Tajikistan; other people suggested getting a taxi across the Pamir Highway. We really didn't want to worry people at home, but we didn't want to make any rash decisions. We decided to continue the journey as planned. The decision came with a commitment to focus on paying extra attention to the kindness and good around us.

Setting off with this intention helped affirm Tajikistan to be the friendly and hospitable country that it is reputed to be. Every smile and wave seemed to motivate us into some of the toughest cycling we had done. By agreeing to make an extra effort to see the goodness around us, I feel like we avoided becoming suspicious of the people we met. Had we not had the intention of looking for the kindness, I imagine I would have been scared or closed off, and instead, even in the wake of unimaginable tragedy, was yet again reminded of how kindness is all around you.

do >

Identify kindness in the wild.

Even the most steadfast optimist needs occasional reassurance that the world is, in fact, good. The signs are ever present if you look for them. Quietly observe the people around you—a kind word here, a helpful act there, community members coming together. You are not alone. Not even close. Jot down what you observe.

learn >

You have studied gratitude for twenty years—what is the definition of "gratitude" that we all should know?

Gratitude is an emotion that helps us hang on to special people in our lives by motivating us to become special people in their lives. We experience gratitude when we realize that someone cares about us more than we had thought. When this happens, they become more valuable to us, so we end up wanting to become valuable to them.

— *Michael McCullough,* PROFESSOR OF PSYCHOLOGY
AT UNIVERSITY OF CALIFORNIA SAN DIEGO

reflect >

THE GIFT OF GRATITUDE

Dear Ryan,

Your unexpected and heartfelt text made me cry tears of joy. I think one of the kindest things anyone can do for another is to express gratitude in very specific terms, and you did this so meaningfully for me. Thank you for understanding that you, your sister, and your brother are always my first priorities. Thank you for acknowledging the sacrifices I make to ensure you all are happy and healthy. And thank you for appreciating the experiences we enjoy together that enrich our lives and help you to become open-minded, purpose-driven people who want to make the world a better place.

You are only thirteen, and I am already in awe of the young woman you are becoming. I am deeply honored and grateful to be your mother.

Beaming you love and light,

— *Momma* (RANA DIORIO,
SAN FRANCISCO, CALIFORNIA)

"The best thing to hold onto in life is each other."

—AUDREY HEPBURN

do >

Send a thank-you text. Unprovoked.

Take a moment right now to think about someone you're grateful for. There's no more immediate way to let them know than for you to send a simple text telling them exactly why you appreciate them.

learn >

"Nice guys finish first." In a series of social experiments, altruists were more likely to gain the respect of their peers, and more likely to be chosen as leaders, than selfish individuals.

(HARDY AND VAN VUGT 2006)

reflect >

I'VE GOT YOUR BACK

In 2001, I was just starting out on my entrepreneurial journey and about to join forces with a seasoned real estate developer. It was a time of excitement and promise mixed with anxiety.

Throughout it all, my business partner checked in on me at the end of each day to make sure I was okay. No matter what disagreements we had or what was said in the heat of the moment, our relationship prospered in large part because of that important gesture. What my father taught me early on resonated often: "The partnership is more important than the deal!"

I had set out to find a partner who could be my mentor. In retrospect, what I probably needed more than anything else was his kindness. Each day, he would help build my skills and confidence. "I have your back, Dean, no matter what" are words I'll never forget. Now, all these years later, I repeat them often to my team members and partners. My associates and employees know that I will ALWAYS support them and their decisions, even when the outcome isn't what we hoped for.

Today, and every day, I try to pay forward what my business partner did for me eighteen years ago.

— *Dean Mendel,* MONTREAL, CANADA

"I think 'Nice guys finish last' is the single most dangerous phrase in the English language."

—DAVID GAZ

do >

Connect with a co-worker— over coffee, tea, or lunch.

Is there someone you work with but don't really know? You may discover that you have more in common than the eight-plus hours a day you spend in the same building. This isn't about networking, or talking shop, or even gossiping. Just get to know each other. Here are a couple conversation starters: What did you want to be when you grew up? If your next vacation was all expenses paid, where would you go? What is a memorable act of kindness you've received?

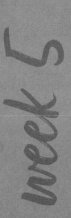

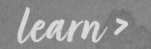

"In a study of 14 countries, **honesty** was universally considered to be an **important virtue**."

(VAN OUDENHOVEN ET AL. 2014)

reflect >

THERE IS KINDNESS IN CLARITY

My first dog was named Frankie and she was seventeen pounds of gray fur, pointy snout, and eerily human blue eyes. One morning, shortly after she turned eight years old, she ignored her kibble. Frankie *always* wanted to eat, so I knew something was up and immediately made an appointment with the vet.

A few blood tests and an ultrasound later, I was standing in the vet's office with tears streaming down my face. There was a growth on her liver and some particularly ominous blood chemistry. The vet outlined the possible diagnoses. When he got to the end, he referred me to a larger veterinary hospital and asked if I had any questions.

"Are there any *good* outcomes here?" I asked.

"I wish you hadn't asked that," he said, sadly. "No."

And just like that, he broke my heart. One clean, quick stroke of honesty that I will always be grateful for. As Frankie went through several more tests, I heard a lot of "maybe"s, a few "if you're lucky"s and a couple of "it's too soon to tell"s. The certainty of that original "no" saved me from a roller coaster of hopes raised and crushed. Frankie died a month later.

The original vet's honesty gave me the clarity I needed at such a tough time. I often think of it and how he didn't *want* to tell me, but he did anyway. The kindest thing was telling me not what I wanted to hear, but what I needed to hear.

—Mollie Goldstein

do >

Consider (and practice) how you can combine honesty and compassion.

Honesty isn't always about the truth versus lies. Sometimes it's about saying what someone doesn't want to hear, but needs to hear. Other times it's about not giving false hope, or false compliments, or saying what is expected. Next time you find yourself needing to talk about something with someone where the truth might hurt, take a moment to reflect on how to deliver it in a way that is thoughtful and empathic.

learn >

"Humble people have the capacity to **laugh at themselves**, which makes them the sort of people **capable of improving**."

—*Professor Mark Alfano,* ASSOCIATE PROFESSOR AT DELFT UNIVERSITY OF TECHNOLOGY AND PROFESSORIAL FELLOW AT AUSTRALIAN CATHOLIC UNIVERSITY

reflect >

Q & A WITH CARLOS NAVARRO

Carlos Navarro is an actor and radio personality.

You have accomplished a lot in your career, but may be best known for The Walking Dead. *How did you land that role?*

It was a dream of mine to get on that series. I spent five years auditioning for different characters before finally being cast. My motto is "to the top, never stop"! In everything, I just want to be the best version of myself.

Wow, that is a lot of effort. How did it feel when you found out they cast you?

The way I imagine anyone would feel when they achieve a big, longtime goal. It was seriously one of the best days of my life.

How long did you stay at your dream job?

I played Alvaro for nine episodes. Then I got a script one week, a few weeks before we were scheduled to shoot, and that's how I found out my character was going to be killed off. I mean, it shouldn't have come as a surprise. It's a zombie show . . . most people die. It's in the title of the series! But it still sucks for any actor to find out, wow, I'm not going to be on the show anymore. I'm not going to be part of that world.

I think a lot of people can relate to that. Did anything help you get through it?

My castmates, who I now think of as family, all called me. None of them had to do that—it's not like I was dying in real life! But they were so sincere and heartfelt in how they sent me off. They are all busy people, but they organized a dinner and toasted me. It was a beautiful moment. On a TV or movie set, everyone works so closely together, you have to be kind. It's a team and a group mentality, and we're still a close crew.

We have to ask: Are zombies kind?

Yes! Zombies don't have to be unkind. They're capable of kindness too.

do >

Book a date with yourself.

Take yourself out to the movies, an art museum, a restaurant, or go to your favorite spot—do an experience that inspires you. Or book a lesson for something you've always wanted to learn. You don't have to be great at it; do it because you enjoy it and keep learning in the process.

learn >

In our research on people's perceptions of kindness, we find that **even the smallest, apparently insignificant acts can have as big an impact** as the larger, apparently more impressive acts.

(KINDNESS.ORG)

week 7

43

THE LASTING WARMTH OF A SIMPLE GESTURE

I'd been waiting for the phone call. It came on a crisp California morning in January. Greg, my thirty-nine-year-old brother, was dying.

"Oh honey," Mom's voice caught, "the hospice nurse thinks it will happen by tomorrow morning."

Even though I'd been with him three months earlier after the stroke caused by a brain tumor, and heard the doctor say, "There's nothing more we can do," it was a shock.

After booking my flight to Illinois, I hurriedly packed and drove a stressful hour on a winding road over the mountains to the airport.

On the plane, I listened to the passengers around me. A mother read to her child, an older couple chatted about their visit to see their first grandchild, two girls behind me giggled. Everything was so normal. I leaned my head back and closed my eyes, willing my tears away.

No food was going to be served on this two-hour flight. My stomach grumbled, betraying the fact that I hadn't even thought about food all morning.

"Excuse me," I said in a faltering voice to a passing flight attendant. She leaned down. "I haven't eaten anything today and am really hungry. I wondered if you have a little bag of peanuts or something." I felt like a small child, not a competent forty-six-year-old woman.

Nodding, she said she'd see if she could find something.

She was gone for a while. I thought she'd forgotten when I saw her walking toward me from the first-class cabin with something wrapped in a napkin. She handed it to me. It was warm. I unwrapped it and found a large freshly baked chocolate chip cookie. I almost cried. It evoked comforting memories of home and family. She smiled as if to say it was no big deal. To me, this small gesture—something she didn't have to do—meant everything.

It's been many years, but I've never forgotten that attendant. She had given me a simple gift that I've carried with me ever since—the gift of kindness, of reaching out to strangers with an open heart, and remembering that everyone has a story.

—*Sandy Raney*, SANTA CRUZ, CALIFORNIA

do >

Be mindful of opportunities to help as they arise.

Planning is wonderful, but opportunities to commit spontaneous acts of kindness are all around us—we're sometimes just too wrapped up in our own worlds to notice. For this kind act, focus on being aware of those around you. See someone wrestling with a heavy bag, in need of directions, or struggling in another, less obvious way? Let the universe guide you to help where you're needed.

learn >

Spending money on others **reduces blood pressure**, with effects comparable to taking blood pressure medication or exercising.

(WHILLANS ET AL. 2016)

47

reflect >

APPRECIATING A STRANGER'S GENEROSITY

One Sunday morning, I went to the local market to look for some fabric. I had recently moved into a new home and was doing a project to cover my couch. In one store, I found the perfect pattern, but they only accepted cash, and I didn't have enough. I asked the retailer to cut me some fabric while I ran to the ATM. A lady standing nearby said, "I will buy it for you." I politely refused. She sweetly insisted and after some back and forth, with her sharing stories about her grandchildren, I accepted her gift.

I used the fabric for cushions that now sit in my living room. Every time I look at them, I am reminded of how generous and giving people can be.

—*Yasmine Hammad,* DUBAI

"If you want to lift yourself up, lift up someone else."

—BOOKER T. WASHINGTON

do >

Pay a stranger's way.

Paying for a stranger's coffee has been known to start a chain reaction. Is the person in front of you short on bus fare? Is someone only getting a few bucks worth of gas? Is someone's parking meter about to run out? You can also anonymously cover the cost of tolls, school lunches, or other incidentals. It's more about the gesture than the amount you spend.

learn >

week 9

"What the world needs more of is **ordinary kindness**—many small actions of caring and connection. Imagine if we just set out every day to do one kind thing or offer one kind phrase or gesture, whether to another person or oneself? We'd have many more sparks of connection illuminating what is beautiful and courageous in humanity. And that is **heroic**."

—*Tara Cousineau,* PHD, CLINICAL PSYCHOLOGIST AT HARVARD UNIVERSITY AND KINDNESS.ORG SCIENTIFIC ADVISOR

51

reflect >

A LIFETIME OF KINDNESS

One of the most subtle examples of kindness I've witnessed is one that has been going on for quite some time. In fact, it began two decades before I was born, when a man named Bob married a woman named Shirley. Bob was a hardworking guy who, at the age of eighteen, left his home in Michigan's Upper Peninsula to do one of the most grunt jobs around—busting frozen coal out of train cars in the winter for a Kalamazoo power plant.

Shirley, who had been married before, was a beautiful woman who came with extra luggage in the form of three rambunctious children. Bob made that family, his. Those kids, his. He watched them become adults, get married, have kids of their own (one of whom was me), who then had kids of their own (none of whom were from me), and watched each one of them mature and grow. One day,

Shirley had a paralyzing stroke. Soon after, Bob retired from his job as superintendent of that same power plant to care for his wife— which he did for fourteen years, until she passed.

Throughout his life, my grandfather has maintained that dedication, treating each member of our family as his own . . . because we are. Has he been perfect? No, he's human. But his love has had a profound impact through the simple, long-lasting acts of kindness in his hard work, uncanny humor, and being there for anyone in need. Even when he hasn't known how to express it or when to show it, he's simply been it.

—*Richard Gretsky,* ORLANDO, FLORIDA/
LOS ANGELES, CALIFORNIA

do >

Count your blessings. Literally.

Being in the present usually serves us well, but every once in a while, it can be good— no, great—to take stock of how far we've come and how much we have. The people we've met, the places we've gone, the obstacles we've overcome . . . Take a few minutes to reflect and write down what you're grateful for.

learn >

Kind acts in the workplace benefit givers and receivers, and are also likely to be **"paid forward,"** leading to even more employee kindness.

(CHANCELLOR ET AL. 2018)

reflect >

Q & A WITH ERIC HUTCHERSON

Eric Hutcherson is an executive vice president and the chief human resources officer for the National Basketball Association. He manages the team that drives the NBA's global workforce strategy, which is built on a commitment to attracting, retaining, developing, and engaging top talent for the NBA and WNBA, NBA G League, and NBA 2K League.

Are there any specific acts of kindness that you try to practice regularly?

I try to end every conversation with "What can I do to be helpful to you?" I say that to almost every person who I see or interact with. In my early days at the NBA, people were skeptical, they thought it was just the typical HR closing line, until I'm still there waiting for the answer—because I really DO want to know. And I really am going to try to help.

Is it easy or hard to consistently be kind in the workplace? As in, does it take a lot of strength?

It can be hard. And to be honest, I think it happens quite often that it is a lot harder than you think. There are plenty of moments when I get it wrong. I say or do something that comes across as insensitive, or I am short with someone. When that happens, I try to acknowledge it and ask how I can fix it.

What advice do you have for someone who is trying to lead with kindness?

Two things: (1) Nobody wants to be led by the productive jerk— the one who is capable and gets stuff done but is a jerk. They may tolerate them because they have to, but they don't want to be around them. (2) Anyone can lead with a hammer. But the best leaders are the ones who can motivate with genuine kindness, even when they themselves have nothing left in the tank. If you can do that, the whole organization will be better. Stay with it, even when it is hard.

do >

Ask if you can help.

Asking *for* help can be hard. But, asking *to* help can be easy. Offer your assistance to colleagues, put the question out on social media, ask a friend or family member. Then spend thirty minutes doing what you can, even if it's only listening—sometimes that is more than enough.

learn >

A meta-analysis of 33 studies suggests that exposure to the **natural environment** can **improve your mood**.

(ROBERTS ET AL. 2019)

reflect >

RECONNECTING WITH MOTHER NATURE

In the summer of 2019, I embarked on a wilderness quest, a twelve-day journey into nature and away from all the comforts of the modern world, including smartphones, clocks, and other technology. Halfway through the experience, I endured the most physically and mentally trying experience of my life (and I've gone through childbirth multiple times!), when I spent four days totally alone, with only a sleeping bag, tarp, and water.

Before I left for my trip, my family had a special dinner planned. My youngest son, Harley, had arranged for everyone to write me letters of encouragement, and I was told to read them the night before I left for the solo portion of my adventure. Those notes saying that they loved and believed in me sustained me through the long, rough days ahead and gave me the courage to keep going whenever I wanted to quit. Because they had faith that I would finish, I knew I would.

The experience, while incredibly difficult, was life-changing, and made me feel reconnected to the planet and everything and everyone on it. My heart cracked open with love and gratitude, and I felt the power and the simple beauty of what a note can do.

Thank you, Harley, Erik, Krystian, Julian, Sam, Chris, and AC, for giving me the encouragement I needed to reconnect with Mother Nature.

—*Tasha Wahl*, SAN DIEGO, CALIFORNIA

do >

Spend some time in nature— a lawn, a park, a forest, or whatever is feasible for you.

If you live in a city or have a long commute, it might seem hard to carve out time to be in nature. But research shows that even spending a few minutes in green spaces can lower your blood pressure and help you feel more connected to the world.

learn >

Forgiving others for past wrongs increases one's positive affect (hope, optimism, and other positive emotions) and **decreases** one's **negative affect** (stress, anxiety, depression).

(LUNDAHL ET AL. 2008)

63

reflect >

THE "F" WORD

My father and I have spent much of my adulthood drifting in and out of estrangement. My mom had a very difficult divorce from my dad, and she expected my siblings and me to cut off contact from him. Sometimes I would agree with her, so angry at what he did (and didn't) do, and sometimes it was just too much of a headache to have them both in my life at the same time. But in other moments, I would want my dad back.

After what was the longest period of no contact with him—my father lived in Reno, Nevada, with his new wife and young kids, and I was in graduate school in Chicago—I finally called him. He didn't even know I was in graduate school. He didn't know I had moved from Seattle to Chicago. I left a message.

He didn't call me back.

Instead, after two weeks, he emailed to tell me that we were finished being father and daughter. Too much time had passed. I was at work when I read his email, walking to a meeting, and I felt myself start to sway as if I would fall. I quickly got myself into the single-stall bathroom and sat on the floor. I texted my boss to tell her I was sick.

I called a confidant, my friend Marcy. I told her, beat by beat, what happened. I asked her what to do. *Was there anything to do?*

Mary said, "Yes, write a letter back. Begin by gently asking for forgiveness."

I replied defensively, "But he never calls me! He's left my life as much as I've left his! And he just told me he didn't want me as his daughter anymore!"

Calmly, she continued, "At the end of the letter, write everything you are grateful for—everything he did for you as a kid." She also told me not to rush it—to respond when I get it right.

I discovered that the act of writing to my father was also the act of forgiving my father. The paragraph I wrote at the end of the letter, where I expressed my gratitude, was what I needed to do to shift my attitude to one of kindness and generosity for my father. A few days later he responded.

Shortly thereafter, I booked a ticket to see him. I didn't have much money at the time, but I made it happen somehow.

I was so excited that I called him from my connecting flight on the Denver tarmac, as I looked out the window at the papercut mountains against the cloudless blue sky.

"I can't wait to see you, Dad."

—*Paula Gilovich,* NORTH CAROLINA

do >

Forgive a past wrong.

Make no mistake: forgiveness is first and foremost a kindness to yourself. Healing doesn't only come with time, but also with intention. Consider how you were hurt, how it affected you, where you are now. Take the first step toward letting go.

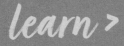

learn >

What is compassion?

The recognition of another's suffering and a desire to alleviate their suffering.

What is compassion for?

Our survival. Compassion is deeply embedded in our DNA. When we care, not only does the recipient of our care benefit, but as importantly, so does the giver. When one is compassionate, those areas of the brain associated with reward and pleasure are stimulated and one's physiology works its best.

—*James R. Doty,* MD, PROFESSOR OF NEUROSURGERY AND FOUNDER AND DIRECTOR OF THE CENTER FOR COMPASSION AND ALTRUISM RESEARCH AND EDUCATION AT STANFORD UNIVERSITY

week 13

reflect >

YOU ARE NOT ALONE

To the Man in the Blue Shirt on the 6 train in New York City,

I was thirty-two weeks pregnant, headed to an ultrasound appointment on the Upper East Side during rush hour. The subway car was packed. I stood, feet throbbing, trying to protect my belly from strangers' elbows. I was exhausted that day, swirling with self-doubt, and silently wishing I had accepted one of my friends' offers to come with me. *How am I going to make it as a single parent? Especially in NYC? Am I really strong enough?* I was urgently and discreetly blinking back tears when you noticed me. You didn't have a seat either, but you shouted out for someone to give me one. Then you parted the masses so that I could reach the open space. Thank you for making me feel a little less alone when I needed it most. We interacted for approximately twenty seconds of my life—but I will never forget you.

—Nicole

"How beautiful a day can be when kindness touches it!"

—GEORGE ELLISTON

do >

Stand, so someone else can sit.

Crowded situations—from a packed bus or subway to a standing-room-only meeting— get us uncomfortably close to strangers. Too often, that's the extent of our connection. Next time, make that contact count and offer your seat to someone else, especially if someone needs it more than you, but even if they don't.

learn >

Just like writing down gratitude improves well-being, writing down the benefits you receive from arguments **makes forgiving easier.**

(MCCULLOUGH ET AL. 2006)

reflect >

KINDNESS ACROSS DIFFERENCE

My wife and I come from different religious backgrounds, and we decided to follow the religion of my wife when raising our children. Our pastor was a fantastic leader, the epitome of what you hope for in representing religion—inclusive, warm, always smiling.

One Sunday, a visiting priest made a very hurtful passing comment to the congregation about my religion.

At the end of Mass, Pat, one of our neighbors, went out of his way to walk over and tell me the priest should not have made that comment and apologized that it took place. Pat didn't draw attention to himself. Just quietly, he wanted to tell me the visiting priest was wrong and the comment shouldn't have happened. To me, this was one of the most meaningful and kind actions that has occurred in my lifetime. I still think about it so many years later. I don't think Pat knows the impact he had that day. But because of what he did, I will always think about Pat—and not the comment. A small act of kindness can have a lifelong impact.

—*Gary S.*, SCOTTSDALE, ARIZONA

"Kindness is the golden chain by which society is bound together."

—JOHANN WOLFGANG VON GOETHE

do >

Reconnect with someone you haven't seen in a while.

Losing touch is possible in the age of social media—maybe more so than ever. Fortunately, so is reaching out again. Make time to connect, either virtually or in person, with that friend from summer camp, former co-worker, or college roommate. That connection can be worth a thousand photos.

learn >

72% of employees think it is important for an employer to **recognize kind acts** in the workplace.

(U.S. CHAMBER OF COMMERCE FOUNDATION 2017)

reflect >

MENTORING WITH THOUGHTFULNESS

親切 (*Shinsetsu*) means "kindness" in Japanese. I was born in Japan but raised in the United States from age two. In 2006, I had been excited to start a job in product support and operations for Google, and I threw myself into it. As my first performance review approached, I was certain that my boss, Denise, would tell me I was doing well. She was something of a legend, having helped launch Gmail.

Instead of praise, though, Denise told me, "Yukari, your self-evaluation is not very detailed and barely highlights what you accomplished these past few months. Why is that?" I explained that in my past jobs, all with Japanese companies, I never had to write about my accomplishments because my boss already knew my work and I was evaluated based on those observations. Writing about my accomplishments felt uncomfortable because it wasn't humble to do so—a big part of Japanese culture. Denise said, "Yukari, you're not working in Japan anymore! Here, you have to be able to express what you've accomplished in order to receive the recognition and rewards you deserve. So, I want you to embrace where you are, and redo it."

To this day, I will never forget Denise's words of encouragement. She was the first female boss that showed me I needed to work hard and, at the same time, stand up for myself in order to be visible and successful in the company. More importantly, Denise demonstrated that you can lead with kindness. Denise chose to be kind and didn't just let me drown in cultural differences. I carry this thoughtfulness with me everywhere and try to pay it forward by leading with kindness一親切に一too.

—*Yukari Pass,* NEW YORK, NEW YORK

do >

Give an occasion-free gift to a loved one or co-worker.

Meaningful gifts aren't as much about getting something as they are about being gotten. Bring in a book your co-worker mentioned wanting to read or surprise a friend with a new pen after she lost her favorite one, and you'll see that it is the thought that really counts.

learn >

Kindness can reduce the negative effects of stress. A 14-day study found that people engaging in prosocial helping had less stress than when the study began.

(RAPOSA ET AL. 2016)

week 16

reflect >

A WELCOME LIKE NO OTHER

Dear Man in the Hawaiian Shirt,

I had been through Penn Station many times as a visitor, but now standing in the middle of the atrium I felt utterly certain I had never seen it so busy. With sweaty palms, I gripped my two suitcases, a handle in each hand, twisting and turning them in confusion with myself. You walked up and somewhat gruffly asked where I needed to go. I stammered I was trying to get to Brooklyn. The A train to the R train, to be exact. In what I now appreciate as a very New York kind of way, you said, "Follow me," and took one of my suitcases and began leading me to the right entrance.

While walking, you shared how you and your husband always love trying to help people with directions. "In a city so big, so overwhelming it's the small things that can help strangers feel more at home."

"Well," I told you, "this actually is now my new home. I just left everything I know, everyone I love, and have moved my life in these two suitcases to live here."

Thank you, sir, for being the tangible arms of New York City that day and welcoming me into them. In a moment of feeling so daunted by my new reality, you reinforced the decision to come. And you will forever be my favorite New York story.

—*J. Galvez,* BROOKLYN, NEW YORK

do >

Let someone go ahead of you in a long line.

Rush, rush, rush. Many days, we can feel like there is so much to do, with not enough hours in the day. And then we have to wait: at the grocery store, at the bank, during rush hour. Let a stranger go first and give them a few unexpected minutes back into their day.

learn >

Kindness is exhibited and celebrated **all around the world**, irrespective of culture. In a survey of 1,063,921 people in 75 countries, **honesty, fairness, and kindness** were among the **most highly endorsed** character traits.

(MCGRATH 2014)

reflect >

AN IMPACTFUL UMBRELLA

Many years ago, I was in Kyoto, Japan. I had been traveling with my parents and had just seen them off to the airport. They had both lived in Japan, so they were my unofficial guides. On my own for the first time, I was wandering around making sense of everything (and feeling rather out of place to be honest), when it started to absolutely pour with rain. I've always taken the view that there is no point in running if it is raining—you might as well just get wet—but suddenly, out of nowhere, a Japanese woman ran up to and pushed an umbrella at me. She bowed and then ran off into the rain. I opened the umbrella and then stood there in this foreign country, marveling at their society. That moment still inspires me to this day—not just for helping others, but for truly doing so with no expectation of return. What greater way to live than as the anonymous Greek proverb says, "A society grows great when old men plant trees whose shade they know they shall never sit in."

—*Didier Elzinga,* MELBOURNE, AUSTRALIA

"Wherever there is a human being, there is an opportunity for a kindness."

—SENECA

do >

Acknowledge someone when they walk into the room.

Too many times, we let the people around us fade into the background of our lives, become part of the scenery. Take some time to see someone, to notice someone— nod hello, make introductions, strike up a conversation, or pay a compliment.

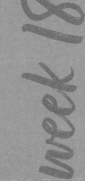

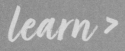

Kindness is contagious.
Kind acts can spread quickly
through social networks.

(FOWLER AND CHRISTAKIS 2010)

Q & A WITH AMY JO MARTIN

Amy Jo Martin, a pioneer of social communication, was the second verified person on Twitter, and with a million-plus following, she originally fell in love with social media because of the positive potential it offered. She's a *New York Times* bestselling author and creator of the podcast *Why Not Now?*

You've championed all things digital for most of your career, and yet, there was a time when you weren't sure it was for you. Tell us about that.

As an early adopter of social media, I originally fell in love with social communication channels such as Facebook and Twitter because of the positive potential they offered. After witnessing the influx of negativity spreading, and experiencing myself how it began to affect my mind every day, I wanted to understand where and how experiencing more kindness online would affect our health. I knew tech wasn't going anywhere, so it was my trying to figure out how tech and I could have a relationship, if at all. One thing has become abundantly clear to me: kindness is critical to both what I put out and what I welcome in.

What's an example of kindness you've experienced digitally?

When I recently gave birth to my first child, Lincoln, he came more than ten weeks early. I was on my way to a mini vacation and went into labor during my layover. We ended up being in the NICU for three months in a city we didn't know very well, with our family states and countries away from us. It was the digital outpouring from people around the world that gave me the energy to navigate such a difficult time. The comments, the positive love and support throughout, the outreach—it was remarkable. And it reminded me daily of the power that kind words online can have.

If you could get everyone around the world to do one act of kindness online, what would it be?

Next time you see any kind of negativity online, anywhere at all, combat it with something positive. With the anonymity that comes with social media, it feels like bullying and plain meanness can be seen everywhere. BUT, I truly believe there are more of us rooting for and wanting to have our social networks be kind places, and it takes each of us doing small acts daily to make it kind for ALL of us.

do >

Respond kindly to a negative comment online.

It may feel like planting a daisy on a garbage heap, but sometimes a gentle or agreeable word can be so unexpected, especially online, that you just might get a response in kind.

learn >

"Compassion is not easy or even natural at first. It is more natural to turn away from pain or want to avoid it. **Compassion takes emotional courage** to face difficult feelings and to respond to another's pain or distress (and to our own)."

—*Tara Cousineau,* PHD, CLINICAL PSYCHOLOGIST AT HARVARD UNIVERSITY AND KINDNESS.ORG SCIENTIFC ADVISOR

reflect >

A GIFT, NOT JUDGMENT, FOR THE MOM OF A SPECIAL NEEDS CHILD

It was the end of a long, tiring workweek and we were celebrating my ex-husband's birthday with the kids. Taking my then three-year-old son out to any public place was always risky, because Anthony is more active than most kids his age—he rarely sits, even with smartphone video games to occupy him—and louder too. He was born deaf and received cochlear implants at age one, but he still has difficulty modulating his voice and volume. He also gets overwhelmed in crowds and noisy places like the chain restaurant we had chosen.

It wasn't long before other patrons noticed. I saw disapproving looks and heads shaking every time my son got up and began racing between the tables, giggling as he dodged us. We took turns chasing after him and even walked with him out in the parking lot to give him a breather, but as soon as we returned, he was back at it. An older couple who had been seated near our table motioned their waiter over and soon got up to leave.

Worse than not being able to just sit and enjoy a meal, I felt the weight of their judgment on me, the mom who couldn't control her child. It was a miserable, helpless feeling.

We asked for the check, ready to call it a night, and prepared to leave an extra-large tip as an apology. But our waiter told us, smiling, that our bill, including tip, had been taken care of. I looked around for someone I knew, but there were only strangers enjoying their dinners. I felt tears of gratitude welling up in my eyes. It wasn't the free meal, but the kinship, the understanding. To this day I have no clue who paid for that dinner, but I suspect it was someone else who knew the struggles of raising a special needs child. I will never forget that night, and the difference that gesture made. Ever since, I have been looking for a similar situation where I can be the hero: An overwhelmed mom, doing her best, being judged in spite of it. And a total stranger who lets her know she isn't alone.

—*Jill Waldbieser*, PENNSYLVANIA

do >

Encourage a friend
who's struggling.

Do you remember a time you didn't
give up because someone gave you the
encouragement you needed? If someone
you know is struggling, having a vote of
confidence in their corner might make
all the difference. Let them know you
are there for them and that you believe
in them.

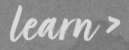

learn >

Spending money on others **makes you happier** than spending money on yourself.

(DUNN ET AL. 2008)

week 20

95

reflect >

TO SPEND, TO SAVE, OR TO GIVE?

Giving to charity was never something that came naturally to me. I largely preferred spending or saving. Then I fell in love with someone for whom "living generously" was nonnegotiable. I wanted the girl, and theoretically, giving seemed like a good thing—how big of an issue could it really be once we were married?

In truth, it wasn't an easy shift. I didn't give cheerfully and was even begrudging about it at times. But eventually, something changed. With every gift that we made, I opened up a little more to the joy that generosity can bring. Now, many years into giving being a normal part of my life, I actually look forward to it. I can honestly say that I prefer giving as much, if not more, as I do saving and spending.

—*Mancel*

"Never believe that a few caring people can't change the world. For, indeed, that's all who ever have."

—MARGARET MEAD

do >

Point, click, and donate to a worthy cause.

There is so much need that trying to decide where to allocate your dollars can leave you feeling overwhelmed and guilt-stricken. It's okay, breathe. You don't need to give away your retirement fund to make a difference. Even small amounts of money can make a huge difference for many great charities. Try using a tool, such as Charity Navigator, to help guide your selection process.

learn >

A study by psychologists at Yale University found that **"a child standing up for another child being bullied"** was considered an exemplary act of heroism.

(KRAFT-TODD AND RAND 2019)

reflect >

FRIENDSHIP AND INCLUSION

I would really like to thank my school friend, Josh. His friendship and kindness mean the world to me. When some people are mean to me because I'm different, Josh is always nice to me and always looks out for me.

—*Alex,* AGE 9, LONDON

"Kindness is truly seeing someone and making them feel less alone."

—LEON LOGOTHETIS

do >

Invite someone to join you in completing a kind act of your choice.

Peer pressure doesn't have to be a bad thing. Inspire someone else to commit an act of kindness! When you lead by example, others may follow, but don't just wait for it. Enlist help with your task and let kindness guide both of you.

learn >

You have to **take care of yourself** in order to take care of others. Try a nap! An experiment by none other than NASA showed that napping improves "physiological alertness and performance."

(ROSEKIND ET AL. 1994)

reflect >

THE POWER OF A POWER NAP

My four siblings and I were blessed with a mom who had the stamina and zeal to rise to any occasion we dropped at her feet. It didn't matter if it was six in the morning or midnight; she would sympathize with our sorry tales or make us feel like a million dollars because a funny story we told her would be met with genuine laughter.

And things just got done—sometimes so fast that I was left wondering if there was a secret helper elf in the house. I have a vivid memory of standing in the kitchen looking for my water glass thinking, "Where on earth did I put it? There's no way Mom washed it already. Isn't she in the basement doing laundry?"

My mom didn't believe in letting dirty dishes wait until morning, but she did believe in naps. Pure and simple. Once a day, she would go upstairs, curl up in bed, and snooze for fifteen minutes or less. When she came back downstairs, she was completely refreshed and raring to go. She was rested and recharged, not stressed, all because of a few minutes of total surrender. It was a thing of beauty.

—*Mary Jo Bartl,* MOLINE, ILLINOIS

"The advice I would give to my younger self is very, very simple: Stop burning the candle at both ends and renew your estranged relationship with sleep. You will be more productive, more effective, more creative, and more likely to enjoy your life."

—ARIANNA HUFFINGTON

do >

Take a nap.

Nodding off at your desk or collapsing from exhaustion doesn't count. Your body knows what it needs, and when. Let it take over one day and lull you into the kind of peaceful, relaxed state that even doing yoga can't. Sleep soundly, awake refreshed.

"**Gratitude** interventions can have **positive benefits** for people in terms of their **well-being**, happiness, life satisfaction, grateful mood, grateful disposition, and positive affect, and they can result in decreases in depressive symptoms."

(DICKENS 2017)

A LETTER TO THE LOVE OF MY LIFE, MY KIND, BEAUTIFUL, AND INSPIRING WIFE, HELLIE

My darling "Gee",

Every day at 13:22, my telephone beeps to remind me of your compassion, kindness, and the beautiful colour of your deep green eyes. It is a daily punctuation that reminds me of the love and bond we shared during our thirty-five years together.

It was December 20, 2018, and we were all in the car—Patrick, Flo, you, and me. I was driving and silent; tears were flowing freely down my cheeks. You had, again, beautifully and majestically rallied as the tumour continued to do its awful work. You were ill, but smiling and laughing with our children—enjoying your family and our complete closeness during the Christmas season. I was stomach-punched by fear and sadness, with thoughts of losing you and the tragedy of our children not continuing to know the most beautiful woman and mother.

Your green eye caught my eye in the rearview mirror. It must have been about 13:20, and in that glimpse, the universe, love. I will carry it forever.

Then a "ping." A message from you. Two images: 🤍🕺

They are everything. They tell me you love me and that we are love. They tell me that you understand and not to feel so sad—you are dancing and you will dance.

It was the kindest, bravest, most poignant, and thoughtful message— one that will always stay with me. It is the essence of you and the essence of us.

We did spend a final Christmas together.

You died in my arms on February 4, 2019.

You walk with me everywhere, but every day at 13:22, we walk and waltz a little closer.

Thank you.

Always and endlessly,

—*Your "Gee"* (MIKE MEANEY,
LYTHAM, LANCASHIRE, UNITED KINGDOM)

do >

Set a daily gratitude reminder on your phone.

Anyone can be intensely grateful when circumstances align in their favor. But cultivating gratitude as a personality trait can take practice. Setting a reminder gives you that opportunity to find and appreciate the joy in life, however small.

learn >

Helping makes you happy.
Our review of 27 experiments found that people assigned to help others were happier than people assigned to help themselves or to do nothing.

(CURRY ET AL. 2018)

reflect >

Q & A WITH SEBASTIAN TERRY

Sebastian Terry is a bestselling author, keynote speaker, and TV host who has inspired hundreds of thousands of people around the world to find happiness and choose kindness. Through his platform, 100 Things, he motivates people to build a bucket list of 100 things that help people to serve others. Sebastian is the national ambassador for Make-A-Wish Australia.

You've written a book, but have you ever been gifted a book that had a big impact on your life?

This may sound odd, but I was once given a book called *Round Ireland with a Fridge*, written by Tony Hawks, an Irish comedian. Essentially, it outlined a guy who lost a bet with his friends and as such had to buy a mini fridge and attempt to literally hitchhike around Ireland with it. The book itself is absolutely hilarious, but more than this, the story unfolded in a way that showcased the kindness of people. From helicopter rides and free accommodation to the simple notion of chasing a goal and building community, this book showed me that people were good and that having fun is imperative to a healthy life.

You've dedicated a lot of your life to spreading kindness, but we know that being kind isn't always easy. When is it hardest for you?

Kindness to others is certainly the hardest when the individual is not being kind to themselves. My whole philosophy of life is that "when oxygen masks fall from the ceiling, we must put ours on first before helping others," and by this, I mean it's really important that we help ourselves first so that we are in a better situation to be of service to others. If I find it hard to motivate or connect with other people, I usually see it as an indicator that I need to be kind to myself first.

Do you have any kind redos?

Thankfully, I've never had any horrible fails when it comes to kindness, but I do think that in the first place, we have to really listen to what is needed rather than impose what we think is needed. A simple example would be the time I tried to help an aspiring singer break into the limelight, but all she really wanted was to break out of her comfort zone and be heard. We worked it out, eventually!

113

do >

Give a book away.

When you finish a good book, give it to someone who you think might like it. Or give it to an unknown recipient. Write a quick note explaining that it is free and leave it in on a park bench, at a doctor's office waiting room, or in a Little Free Library (freelibrary.org). It's not littering; it's "literaturing."

learn >

"**Heroism** serves as a culturally specific, group-beneficial ideal; it is a quality that evokes awe, becomes integrated into the stories of our cultural heritage, and serves to inspire others to engage in similar acts of **self-sacrifice for the greater good.**"

—*Gordon Kraft-Todd,* PHD, POSTDOCTORAL FELLOW, DEPARTMENT OF PSYCHOLOGY, BOSTON COLLEGE

reflect ›

BONDED OVER KIDNEYS

It was a typical day at work until I overheard a conversation. My boss was talking to a friend about someone with a failing kidney who couldn't find a match for a kidney donation. And to this day, I don't know why, but something went through my mind and I wondered if there was a way I could help. I'm probably not who you imagine when you think of someone donating a kidney to a stranger; I'm a simple man who loves skateboarding and tattoos and spending time with my wife and two boys.

I went into the room and apologized for eavesdropping, but asked for more info on what was wrong with my boss' friend. I spoke to my family and spent time learning as much as I could about what it's like to donate a kidney. The more I learned, the more I realized the incredible need: every day, thirteen people die waiting for a kidney. When I felt armed with knowledge and support, I knew I was ready to take the next step. I wanted to meet this man to know if he was a generally good person. We met, and I knew immediately he was someone I could give up an organ for, despite not really knowing him.

Once I knew that I wanted to do it, we moved quickly. After a week of intense testing, we discovered I was actually a perfect match. Crazy. Seriously crazy. The procedure itself was easy and painless—my scars are barely visible. Nothing about my life really changed, but everything about his did. He's now a grandfather to two kids. He's alive.

And while all of this might sound crazy or hard, all I ask is that you're willing to learn more. I would never have pictured myself doing it before, but everything changed for me once I was educated on it.

—*Max Suarez,* QUEENS, NEW YORK

do >

Learn how to become an organ donor.

Lots of people dismiss the idea outright, but there are several different ways to donate. It doesn't have to be a kidney; bone marrow and umbilical cord blood are among the options as well. And don't forget about posthumous donation: it can be as simple as checking a box when you renew your driver's license. Take time to find options near you; no matter where you are, there is likely need.

learn >

Kindness is in our genes— according to several studies conducted over the past decade, kindness has a genetic component.

(STEGER ET AL. 2007)

reflect >

GIVING THE GIFT OF TIME
AND KNOWLEDGE

In 1995, I spent the summer of my junior year in college working at the National Institutes of Health in a lab doing cancer research. I also had the opportunity to get experience in the medical clinic and sit in grand rounds, the weekly meeting of physicians and students, where they discussed interesting cases. I knew nothing! I would sit in the meeting listening to the foreign words and see the intimidating white coats and try to absorb some of what was happening around me.

At my third meeting, one of the intimidating physicians in a white coat looked over at me and said, "You have any idea what non-small cell lung cancer is?"

"Not really," I replied.

He told me to stay after the meeting, and then he sat down with me for an hour and explained what happened in that meeting and what a number of the technical terms meant. The physician recognized I was likely intimidated and didn't understand. He used his stature not to make me feel less than, but to bring me up.

His kindness opened up a huge door for me. First, I spent the rest of the summer with a much better understanding of what was happening. Second—and more important—it taught me that I was actually surrounded by people who would be kind and helpful if I reached out. The experience made me confident to speak up when I don't understand and fearless to reach out to strangers for help. While not everyone may respond kindly, most people will, and you just have to find them. This physician, Dr. Carmen Allegra, has remained a friend to me some twenty-plus years later.

—Anne Wojcicki, CO-FOUNDER AND CEO OF
23ANDME, SAN FRANCISCO, CALIFORNIA

do >

Thank someone who made a difference in your life.

No one gets anywhere without help. There are probably several people in your past who helped you at a crucial juncture. Teachers and bosses, sure, but also casual acquaintances you may not have kept in touch with, who never realized just how much of an impact they had on you. Look them up and drop them a note to let them know they mattered, and exactly how.

learn >

You've spent a decade studying smiles. Isn't smiling just smiling?

There are many different types of smiles—felt smiles, social smiles, masked smiles, etc. However, all include the innervation of the zygomaticus major muscle. Many smiles are signals. They are for communicating subjective positive affect and prosocial intentions. Because our facial expressions are tied to our emotional states, they can increase the credibility of promises to act prosocially.

—*Dr. Lawrence Ian Reed,* CLINICAL ASSISTANT PROFESSOR AT NEW YORK UNIVERSITY

reflect >

ARE YOU SMILING AT ME?

I was walking down the street, noise-canceling headphones on, eyes straight ahead, zero interest in engaging with anyone until I reached my destination.

As I walked, I caught a glimpse of a smile on the face of an elderly man as we passed each other heading in opposite directions. Was he smiling at me? Huh. Back to my podcast.

A few minutes later, it happened again. Another smile. What the heck? Why were these strangers smiling at me? This was not the norm.

Then the podcaster cracked a joke and I laughed out loud. OMG. My focus moved from my podcast world to reality, and I was hit with a very clear realization: I must have been smiling randomly while listening. Strangers weren't smiling at me. I was smiling AT THEM. They were just smiling back. Hmm. It was actually kinda nice.

—*Grayson,* SAN FRANCISCO

"The shortest distance between two people is a smile."

—VICTOR BORGE

do >

Try a smile experiment.

No one likes being told to smile, especially by a stranger. But smiling does affect you and those around you in ways you may not expect. How do your facial expressions reflect your mood? Are you smiling when you don't feel like it? Hiding it when you do? What happens if you change that? How are people reacting? And most importantly, how does it make you feel? You don't have to go full Cheshire-Cat mode, but you might enjoy a real, unforced smile— your own, or someone else's—more after this experiment.

learn >

More than **one-third** of people over the age of 60 say they **are lonely**.

(ANDERSON AND THAYER 2018)

reflect >

A RESTAURANT THAT SERVED DIGNITY

To the Staff at Noodle & Sushi Delight in Elk Grove Village, Illinois,

I want to serve up a hearty helping of thanks—for your food, service, and atmosphere (which are all exceedingly good), but mostly I want to thank you for the kindness and respect you have shown my parents over the years.

In a world where so many people ignore or marginalize the elderly, the genuine interest you took in my mom and dad during our recent visit absolutely floored me. It was a joy to see their faces light up when they saw you. From your warm smiles and heartfelt greetings when they walked through the front door to the extra almond cookies you slipped in their "doggie" bags when they left, your kindness made a huge difference and it mattered more than you will ever know.

My parents always looked forward to talking with you during their weekly visit to your restaurant. Please know that they were both sad to say goodbye to you when they decided to move 350 miles west, so they could be closer to me, my husband, and our daughter. The last time they saw you, they were in a bit of shock—they had not expected that their home would sell as quickly as it did. They had just over a month to take care of all the moving details.

Because you took the time to really get to know them, I wanted you to know how they are doing. They are champs. They have checked the items off their to-do list and are settling in. They have even found some new restaurants that offer tasty food. But the nourishment they received from you went far beyond what was on the plates you brought to the table. You gave them dignity and a sense of belonging—soul-satisfying side dishes for which we are all incredibly grateful.

—*Cheryl O'Donoghue,*
the Daughter of Don and Diane

do >

Spend quality time with an elderly relative, neighbor, or resident of a retirement community.

Imagine having years of experience and dwindling opportunities to share it. Seek out someone of postretirement age and engage them—ask for advice, get their life story, share in their experiences. Do it while they're still here to appreciate it, and while you're still able to benefit from it.

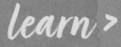

learn >

"**Generosity** is a willingness to help those in need **without expecting to be repaid.**"

—*Athena Aktipis,* PHD, CO-DIRECTOR OF THE HUMAN GENEROSITY PROJECT

reflect >

ONE SMALL ACT CHANGED
THE COURSE OF MY LIFE

I had come to Fort Lauderdale, Florida, from Peru in 1981, with everything I owned stuffed in a small suitcase. I was eighteen, and determined to build a meaningful life for myself. I bought a used ten-speed bike and found a job at a restaurant, but it didn't take long to realize that I needed a high school degree. While I had attended school here and there, I had never graduated. So, I signed up for the GED exam. The only problem: the testing location was twenty miles away.

On the day of the test, I woke up early to start the hour-and-a-half bike ride. Halfway there, it started to downpour. By the time I arrived at the center, the door was shut and there was a sign on the door that read, "No one will be allowed to enter once the exam begins." I was devastated. I noticed a silver-haired gentleman at the front of the room and frantically waved him over. When he opened the door, he said, "I'm sorry, son, the test has already begun."

I told him I had ridden my bike twenty miles in the rain because this test was so important to me. He sensed my urgency and made an exception, letting me in. That day, I passed the exam. Getting my GED helped, but meeting that man is what really changed my life.

That man's name was Cliff and he became a very important person in my life. I stayed after the exam and he ended up becoming first a mentor, then a father figure to me. He inspired me to join the military and to pursue all the dreams I had when I first arrived in this country.

Cliff was the only father I ever really had—a man that my children came to call Grandpa Cliff.

—Sean San Roman

do >

Turn your no into a yes.

The frenetic pace of modern life can trigger a desperate need to safeguard what little time, energy, and space we have for ourselves. The irony is that doing so sometimes shuts us off from the very experiences that help us grow or the simple ways we can help each other. Take one week to open your mind, heart, and eyes, and say yes to opportunities or small favors you normally wouldn't.

learn >

Research has found evidence that play at work is linked with less fatigue, boredom, stress, and burnout in individual workers. Play is also positively associated with **job satisfaction**, a sense of competence, and **creativity**.

(PETELCZYC ET AL. 2018)

reflect >

Q & A WITH MICHELLE GARSIDE

Michelle Garside is co-founder of Soul Camp, a completely transformative sleepaway camp for adults, and Soul Camp Creative, a full-service marketing agency devoted to working with conscious companies and brands that are positively impacting the planet. Michelle and her companies have been featured in *O, The Oprah Magazine, Travel + Leisure, Fitness, Women's Health, Parents, Fortune,* and *Forbes,* and on *Good Morning America* and *ABC News.* She's been involved with kindness.org since day one as an avid volunteer.

You've built a business around nurturing people's souls. How does kindness play a role?

Kindness is seeing the humanity in each and every stranger. It's looking at people through the lens of unity rather than separateness. It's recognizing that we are all in this thing—life—together. It's about operating in a way that invites strangers to feel better in your presence. It's understanding that everyone is struggling in their own way, and everyone, EVERYONE, wants to feel connected, accepted, and not alone. It's living a life that welcomes community over competition. And it's really getting that it starts with you—kindness must first be an inside job.

How do you cultivate and practice kindness in your life?

Vulnerability is key. I try to share struggles. Lead with my heart. See others in their greatness instead of in their lack. Believe in the goodness. Hunt for the beauty. And I try to always remember that at the end of the day, we are all just ants on a spinning ball in space.

When is kindness the hardest for you?

When we are in a state of self-hating, isolation, and aren't able to be kind to ourselves. That's when I think it is near impossible to be authentically kind to others. Kindness, acceptance, and connection must first begin within.

What's the best way to shower yourself with kindness?

Dress in all the colors of the rainbow, roll down a hill, laugh yourself silly, play hooky once in a while. Life is short, so make it fun!

do >

Play! Do something fun with your kids or something that gets you back to the kid you used to be.

Remember when you could while away a day without a to-do list, when you were content just to explore the world around you or create one in your imagination? Don't let adulting erase that. Having pressures and challenges makes finding the wonder and simple pleasures in life that much more essential.

learn >

Self-compassion—the "tendency to **treat oneself kindly** in the face of perceived inadequacy" —is an important predictor of well-being.

(NEELY ET AL. 2009)

THE CARE PACKAGE

It's December 18, two days before I am done with my first semester of graduate school at Columbia University in New York City, two days before I can be reunited with my husband, who still lives in California. My eyes sting from sleep deprivation and my head throbs like I've been hit with a brick. *How are you possibly going to finish everything on time?* I think to myself, as another wave of panic washes over me.

After hours of tortuous paper writing, I receive a text message from a friend who lives in Texas. It feels good to hear from her. She tells me to head to the entrance of my apartment building. When I arrive on the ground floor, there is a delivery man waiting for me.

"Are you Elizabeth?" the delivery man asks, holding a brown paper bag in his hands.

"That's me," I say, with as much enthusiasm as I can muster. He hands me the brown paper bag. Inside, there are three delicious-smelling homemade bone broths and a bright smoothie.

Another text from my friend pops across my phone:

"I believe in you!!!! You're working toward fulfilling your dream life and are a huge inspiration to me every day. Just wanted to send you some care while you're making the final push this week! You are amazing!"

The tears pour down my cheeks. It's as if the reality of everything I have sacrificed by moving across the country to chase after my dreams finally sinks in. Amid all the stress, I hadn't given myself permission—until now—to accept that things have not been easy.

As I wipe the snot from my nose and rub my tired eyes, I am overcome with gratitude. Gratitude for the nourishing food. Gratitude for my loving friend. And most of all, gratitude for the four powerful words: "I believe in you."

—*Elizabeth Su,* **NEW YORK, NEW YORK**

do >

Treat someone without even being there.

When used correctly, technology can bring us closer together. Case in point: You can order food for someone (hungry friend, college student during finals, new mom) from thousands of miles away. Pick a person who you think could use some nourishment and ask what they are craving this week.

learn >

Having self-compassion after a mistake or moral transgression **increases motivation** to make amends and avoid the same mistake in the future.

(BREINES AND CHEN 2012)

reflect >

FORGIVENESS MAY TAKE TIME

I recently went to my college ex-boyfriend's wedding. When I was his girlfriend, I was horrible to him—immature, bratty, and selfish. We broke up in a spectacular fashion on New Year's Eve, when I confessed that I had been cheating on him. His family hated me afterward.

Years later, as I matured, I realized I owed them all an apology. I wrote a handwritten letter to his parents and emailed his brother. My ex, who I had become friends with again, told me his mother was so touched that she cried and carried the letter around for weeks.

His brother was different. He wrote back immediately to tell me he didn't forgive me. I knew to let him have the last word, rather than try and defend myself. He was still angry and I had to accept that.

So, when the time came to attend my ex's wedding, I was nervous. I hadn't seen any of these people in years. But that night, I had the most loving conversations with each of them. They were as genuinely happy to see me as I was them.

I had apologized, but they had to forgive me in their own time. I knew enough to leave them alone. I was sincere in my apology and let it go. Life marched on. As time passed, I became a very small part in a distant memory, so when we saw each other at my ex's wedding, it was really beautiful.

—*Domenica Ruta,* NEW YORK, NEW YORK

do >

Apologize from the heart.

Admit you are wrong, first to yourself,
then to the other person. It could have
happened long ago, or very recently. It
could be something small, or it could mean
everything. It doesn't matter. Be direct;
don't make excuses. Tell them you know
what you did, and you're sorry. Understand
this doesn't guarantee forgiveness. And
that's okay. This is about you and doing the
right thing.

learn >

Joshua (Josh) Ogure is the project coordinator for the Map Kibera Trust and a citizen reporter. In 2017, he led our team of eight citizen scientists investigating kindness in Kibera, Kenya, a neighborhood in Nairobi that is considered to be the largest urban slum in Africa. That research found that kindness in Kibera shares many of the features of kindness that have been identified in other communities. In particular, kindness is closely linked to action and virtue. However, Kiberan communities were found to possess a conception of kindness that is strongly associated with saving and protecting people from violence.

week 33

THE DAY YOU SAVED MY LIFE

Here is a letter from Josh thanking a friend for an act of kindness that we would describe as an act of heroism.

Dear John Paul,

It's been twelve years since that fateful day—the day you saved my life in Naivasha during the postelection violence in 2007. I was stuck inside, surrounded by hundreds of militia who had already killed my neighbor. You came from nowhere, with a small stick in your hands, to rescue me. I heard my neighbor cry for help, until she was murdered by them. I was sure I was next. You called me and I covered myself with a blanket so the enemy wouldn't hear. You told me you were coming and said to get ready to run to you. You were already safe at the police station, but you snuck out, and you and your two cousins risked your own lives to save me. I couldn't believe it when we reached safety. You and God are the reason I am alive today. Thank you so much, brother. Thank you so much, friend. I will never forget you.

Yours truly,

—*Josh* (JOSHUA OGURE)

"You cannot do a kindness too soon, for you never know how soon it will be too late."

—RALPH WALDO EMERSON

do >

Take time to get informed about an important social issue.

Next time you're online, search with purpose: find out more about a political candidate running for office, or a recent headline about a global crisis, even an issue in your local community. We are all citizens of this world and being educated is a moral imperative.

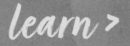

learn >

"**Generosity** is part of human nature."

—*Athena Aktipis,* PHD, CO-DIRECTOR OF THE HUMAN GENEROSITY PROJECT

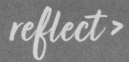

THOUGHTS FROM AN
ALMOST CENTENARIAN

Since I was a little girl, I have memories of what it meant to be a good neighbor. When I was five or six, my dad was very sick and we lived in a third-floor apartment. We lived there for twenty-one years and there is so much to remember. But one of my earliest memories is of a woman living in my building who also ran the grocery store below us. Every day she'd give us a little bit of food because times were so hard. She'd be generous with what she had. I was a little girl but I will never forget the small ways she loved our family.

And now here I am, ninety-six years old, living in a new place, a new state. With the help of my daughters and kind neighbors, I have been able to live alone in my home of forty-five years. And these neighbors, here, too—we've been through so much together. They know I don't walk very well, and every day, they bring my newspaper up to my door for me. And I'll bake them a cake, which is still a favorite thing of mine to do. And that's the beautiful thing— the giving and taking in the smallest of gestures to show up for your neighbor.

—*Ellen Conforti*

do >

Get to know your neighbors.

Invite them over for lemonade or tea, or bake them a cake (never underestimate the community-building power of carbs). Even if you don't bake, think of another way to get to know the folks next door, upstairs, or across the way. Neighbors are the spare-key holders, snow shovelers, and vacation-mail collectors of the world—and you're one of them, wherever you live. Be a good one.

"When I was young, I admired clever people. Now that I am old, I admire kind people."

—ABRAHAM JOSHUA HESCHEL

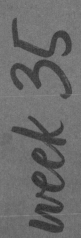

learn >

There are **5.25 trillion pieces** of plastic debris in the ocean.

(PARKER 2015)

reflect >

THE LAZY LITTERER

I've never been a litterbug, but I have been a lazy litterer. You know, the type who might litter around the trash can when the trash ball doesn't quite make it in. Four out of five times, I'd go back and pick it up, but there was always that one time when I thought, *Eh, close enough, someone else will get it*. Those times almost always happened at work, when throwing paper into the little, overfilled wastebasket by the bathroom door. I'd think, *Move on, I've got big important things to do*. But then the guilt would follow. I'd think about all the people who share the "I'm too busy" lazy litterer attitude, and how each and every little piece of litter could really pile up into someone else's headache. Then one time, finally the guilt was too much, and I couldn't pay attention in my next meeting. That was it. I went back to the bathroom, picked up all the little paper towel trash balls, and vowed to never be a lazy litterer again.

—*Sergio Navarro*, NEW YORK, NEW YORK

"The time is always right to do what's right."

—MARTIN LUTHER KING JR.

do >

Clean up someone else's act.

Keep a plastic bag in your car, handbag, or backpack so you can dispose of any litter you find as you go about your day. It doesn't matter that it isn't your trash, because eventually, it becomes everyone's trash. Let's make the world a cleaner, more beautiful place.

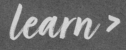

learn >

Kindness **improves the well-being** of both the giver and the receiver.

(PRESSMAN ET AL. 2015)

_ week 36

159

reflect >

KINDNESS IS A UNIVERSAL LANGUAGE

Dear Cristi,

It has been almost three years since we first met and I often think about that day and wonder, *What if I had decided to do something else instead?* On that day, I was the most lost that I had ever felt and was desperately looking for someone to call my friend. As you know, I had moved from Mumbai, India, and hadn't met a single friend, which is a major thing when you are fifteen. I saw a Facebook post for an event, but I had misunderstood it. I thought I was showing up for a social gathering, not a job interview for an events organizer!

You offered me the job, but gave me so much more than that. I barely knew any Romanian and you were patient. You have taught me so many things. You helped me believe in myself. Practicing Romanian with you and the rest of the team is a huge part of why I was able to pass the big exam to finish high school.

You're now my best friend, and I am forever grateful and thankful to you that you decided to be kind when you could have been anything else. I hope I can be a friend that you can continue to trust and be proud of.

With love,

—Tushar, BUCHAREST, ROMANIA

"A warm smile is the universal language of kindness."

—WILLIAM ARTHUR WARD

do >

Share your knowledge with someone.

Teaching as a profession is a calling. But even if you're not a teacher, odds are good that someone else can benefit from the wisdom currently locked in your head—whether that wisdom is about the proper height of a bike seat or how to ask where the bathroom is in French. Sharing your skills is a good way to connect with others and shine a little light of knowledge in the world.

learn >

82% of surveyed youth felt a personal responsibility to **promote kindness and positivity** in the world.

(CASSANDRA 2016)

reflect >

FROM NEIGHBORS TO FRIENDS

After eight years as a researcher who works in the field of kindness, one particular act of kindness stands out as quite powerful and memorable. In a graduate class on social and emotional learning, I had my students plan and enact a series of kind acts. Students were instructed to stretch themselves and reach beyond friends and family when identifying the recipients of their acts of kindness.

A mature student in the class described living in the same condominium complex for nine years, having never spoken to her neighbors. They avoided eye contact in the parking lot and never acknowledged one another when their paths crossed. For her assignment, she put together a gift basket of homemade treats for each of her next-door neighbors. She described the trepidation she felt knocking, with a trembling hand, on their doors to deliver the gift basket. She included a note acknowledging that they'd fallen into a pattern over the years of ignoring one another and she was seeking to change that.

To her surprise and delight, her simple act of kindness changed the interaction pattern between her and her neighbors. Her neighbors were overjoyed to receive homemade treats and appreciated my student taking the first step. Social invitations followed for barbecues and to a bar mitzvah! This student's act of kindness changed how she felt about where she lived by creating community and connection to others within her condominium complex.

—*J.T. Binfet,* PHD, KINDNESS RESEARCHER, UNIVERSITY OF BRITISH COLUMBIA

do >

Learn the name of a person you see regularly (mail carrier, neighbor, store clerk) but still don't know.

Real life doesn't have a "tag" feature, so introduce yourself. When someone tells you their name, repeat it, remember it, and use it. Humanizing the people around us can make the world seem a little smaller and closer and friendlier for everyone.

learn >

Being kind to yourself—
**treating yourself with
compassion**—reduces the
negative emotions people
feel when they reflect on
difficult experiences.

(LEARY ET AL. 2007)

reflect >

A LETTER TO MYSELF

Dear Genevieve,

We've known each other my whole life . . . and I can't believe I've never taken the time to thank you.

Thank you, first, for so many memories. Remember in first grade when you realized how important humor is? Remember when you almost drowned multiple times, and you told me there are just some things we can't control? When you encouraged me when I felt overwhelmed or scared about something that meant take the leap? When we took a step back and realized, wow, so lucky, we officially have too many overwhelmingly good life experiences and important realizations to remember each specific one. But you still insisted that we try to keep track of them in writing (in notebooks and in your phone notes!) . . .

I've looked up to your open-mindedness, spontaneity, and free-spiritedness during my best times, and I've relied on your emotional strength, compassion, and gut instincts through my toughest times. Thank you for always keeping me updated about the exciting things you learn, taking me out to your favorite new places, or just staying in and reading with me, watching TV shows, doing nothing.

It's been easier to show my frustration with you instead (I hope you can forgive me for that)—frustration about your tendencies to get overemotional and be moody, when you're unable to express your feelings, when you shut down in self-pity, and how you're not that great with time or following through with everything we try to plan . . .

But, you constantly remind me that there is more to learn, more people to meet, more thoughts to think, more places to go, more experiences to have . . . I admire you, and the qualities I admire about you exist within myself. Thank you for everything. It's comforting to know you will always be there because you're me.

—XO

do >

Give future you a boost.

Imagine the kind of elation you get from
discovering a five-dollar bill in the pocket of a
coat you haven't worn in a while. Jot down a
good memory or a text that made you laugh
hysterically, or print out a photo from a great
trip. Tuck these into seldom-used locations—
your car's center console, nightstand drawer,
or even that same coat pocket. You'll get a
smile when you least expect it—but when you
just may need it most.

learn >

People assigned to **spend money on others were happier**—and were rated as happier by observers—than those assigned to spend money on themselves.

(AKNIN ET AL. 2014)

reflect >

QUIET KINDNESS

Although I'd become an expert at stretching a dollar, sometimes it came down to this: Should I pay the electric or water bill?

My Aunt Betty and Uncle Frank lived pretty far away, but they made a point of coming to visit my daughters and me as often as they could. Uncle Frank would always check to see if anything needed fixing. He'd tighten a door hinge, check my tires, and more. Aunt Betty filled the house with laughter, love, baked goods, and the latest family updates.

During one visit from them, my heart was already full from everything. Then Uncle Frank asked if he could have my car keys "to see how it was running." The next day when I got in my car with the girls, my gas tank was full. I cried. My uncle had taken my car to the gas station, filled it up, and washed it. Times were hard, so the gas was great (and needed), but it was so much more than that. He was a man of few words, a gentle giant, and he made me feel supported without ever making me feel less than.

—*Diane Southard,* FLORIDA

"The smallest act of kindness is worth more than the grandest intention."

—OSCAR WILDE

do >

Earmark a five-dollar bill in your wallet for random acts of kindness.

Mark it with a sticky note as a reminder and tuck it into a separate part of your wallet. Then, when a moment arises, use your designated kindness cash to help someone else in need. Replace the bill and repeat.

learn >

A meta-study of 29 studies found mindfulness-based therapy (MBT) to be an **effective treatment** for various psychological problems, particularly for **reducing stress**, depression, anxiety, and distress.

(KHOURY ET AL. 2015)

week 40

175

reflect >

Q & A WITH DR. MEGAN JONES BELL

Dr. Megan Jones Bell is chief science officer at Headspace, a leader in the field of digital health and a visionary in making mental health care more effective, affordable, and accessible to all populations. Megan leads the company's science team, which focuses on developing evidence-based interventions and clinically validating the benefits of Headspace.

How do you see kindness and meditation overlapping?

Mindfulness meditation is the practice of cultivating awareness and compassion for oneself and for those around us. So naturally, kindness is a key part of meditation practice. In order to be kind to others, we must first learn how to be kind to ourselves. By taking time out for ourselves to practice meditation, we are developing the skills to be kind to ourselves. At first, it might not be immediately obvious how sitting in isolation and focusing on the breath can benefit other people, but when we're training the mind to be kinder, less judgmental, and more understanding, it makes sense that meditation can have a positive effect on our relationships and the world around us. In feeling awareness and compassion for oneself, we feel awareness and compassion for others.

How have you seen meditation translate to real-world impact?

There are immediate, short-, and long-term benefits of practicing meditation, and we're just at the beginning of understanding how far-reaching these benefits can be. In twenty-three published studies in some of the leading peer-reviewed journals, we've shown that meditation can lead to favorable outcomes, like reduced stress, improved focus, increased compassion, and decreased aggression.

do >

Give meditation a go.

Sure, it can seem strange or daunting if you haven't done it before, and hard to maintain even if you have. The solution for novices and experts is the same, though: practice. The benefits of committing to a fifteen-, five-, or even one-minute daily practice are real, and you'll almost immediately feel them. Also, because meditation is not one-zen-fits-all, you can find an approach that works for you, whether it's a walking, silent, or guided meditation, or some other style.

Two-year-olds prefer puppets who "win," but **not those who win by using aggression**—in which case they prefer the puppet who "lost."

(THOMAS ET AL. 2018)

week 41

179

reflect >

FINDING GRACE WHEN SOMEONE IS UNKIND

One day, I was heading to my car when a complete stranger said something cruel right to my face. I won't repeat it because I don't want to give those negative words more power than they deserve. When it happened, I was shocked. In a daze, I got into my car and that's when I started to feel furious that I hadn't said something back to him.

How dare he judge me like that. It wasn't even true! I wanted to find him and put him in his place—maybe even say some unkind things back to him. That would be fair, right?!

While I drove, I reflected on my rage and whether it was doing me any good. I always wanted to be the person who had a witty comeback. I'd be disappointed in myself when I could only think of the "right" thing to say hours later. As I thought about it, my hands tensely gripping the steering wheel, I realized that if I had reacted with anger, it would have just added to the unkindness that man had shown. I realized that no matter what is done to me, I have control in how I respond.

From then on, I will always choose kindness. Nothing can ever take that choice away from me.

—*Heather Brown,* BOURNEMOUTH, UNITED KINGDOM

"In the long run, the sharpest weapon of all is a kind and gentle spirit."

—ANNE FRANK

do >

Choose kindness, even in the face of its opposite.

It is tempting—even instinctual—to respond defensively to an attack. To curse out the driver who cut you off or shoot a dirty look at the person who stepped on your foot. Instead, pause, reflect, and give the benefit of the doubt. Channel empathy and understanding. And realize that this is but a single, small moment in your otherwise glorious life. Respond with compassion until it becomes your new instinct.

week 42

"Empathy" and **"helping others"** are among the most important traits parents want to teach their kids. Families may differ, but they share common values on parenting.

(PEW RESEARCH CENTER 2014)

reflect >

KINDNESS IS A MUSCLE

When I think about the transformative power of kindness, I think of Johanna (not her real name), the fiery first grader who challenged me unlike any other during my first year teaching. Johanna was growing up in an environment that required a tough outer shell and on-call aggression.

I realized she would need help learning what kindness looked like. We would need to practice. So, I launched a class-wide kindness project to build everyone's kindness muscle.

One day during lunch, a small girl tripped and bumped into Johanna from behind. Like a reflex, Johanna whipped around and puffed her chest, but then caught my eye.

"Remember, we're choosing kindness," I said gently but firmly.

Johanna's response forever changed my understanding of kindness, and of teaching.

Frustrated with herself, she quietly said, "Oh! . . . I keep forgetting."

Choosing kindness was so radically different than the script she had been given, she didn't just need to practice doing it, she had to practice remembering it.

And this is when I saw the change. Once Johanna trusted it was safe, she began to put down her armor and wade into the world of kindness. As she did, she became a different student before my eyes. Sensitive and tender. Highly creative. Socially gifted. Joyful.

For Johanna, kindness was a muscle that had never been allowed to develop. For me, it was like watching a butterfly struggling through its cocoon before flying away, free.

—*Rebecca Reed,* ORLANDO, FLORIDA

do >

Talk to a child about kindness.

Start the conversation with simple questions. What does kindness mean to you? How does it feel when you are kind to someone? How does it feel when someone is kind to you? What acts of kindness do you think the world needs more of? If you don't have kids, don't worry, this is also a great table talk with adults during brunch or over dinner!

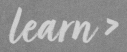

Kindness **reduces social anxiety** in the giver.

(TREW AND ALDEN 2015)

187

GETTING EMPATHY FROM AN UNEXPECTED SOURCE

When I was twelve, my class took a school trip to France. I had looked forward to it for months, and was excited about traveling by train—so excited that when the train arrived I ran on and grabbed a table seat for my friends and me.

It was only as the train began to roll out of the station that I noticed a suitcase that looked remarkably like mine sitting on the platform. The bottom of my stomach dropped out as it dawned on me that I had left everything I packed for the trip behind. It didn't help that my entire class of fellow twelve-year-old boys immediately heard what I'd done and ragged on me about it for a good hour, the sound of their laughter echoing down the carriage.

My unlikely ally in all this was my math teacher, Mr. Furlong-Brown. I feared him, but respected him. He stuck up for me, and even ended up taking me clothes shopping so I at least had clean pajamas for the trip (although they were a pretty awful zebra-striped pattern).

I was hugely embarrassed, but he never added to that by making a big deal out of it. Later, he even made a point of saying in front of the entire class how well I'd dealt with a bad situation, and that they could all learn a thing or two from me.

The truth was that I had been an idiot, and he helped me out more than he had to. It was an act of kindness that has stuck with me for over thirty years. Thank you, Mr. Furlong-Brown.

—*Steven Byrne*, MANCHESTER, UNITED KINGDOM

do >

Change your bad mood with a good deed.

Sometimes when we're feeling down, anxious, or even mad, the last thing we want to do is be kind. But give it a try and see what happens. Next time you are feeling less than great, pick a small act of kindness, do it with intention, and note how you feel afterward.

learn >

9 in 10 young people believe performing small acts of kindness will help **make the world a better place.**

(CASSANDRA 2016)

reflect >

GIVING CREDIT WHERE CREDIT IS DUE

Dear Tom,

I wonder if you'll remember this.

It was years ago, on set, just before we wrapped season two. We were shooting in "dad's" cavernous, creepy penthouse set and there was an issue with blocking. Being that it was a long scene with maybe five other actors, our positioning was crucial, but I had a solution: a change in how we entered the scene, which would allow for a smoother transition to the action later. But, it wasn't that the director waved off my suggestion as I was saying it; what got me was when, a few minutes later, realizing it was a good idea, he turned to you and gave the credit.

Yes, an insignificant moment in the grand scheme of things. My ego didn't need the recognition and the scene finally worked, but it stung. Mostly because it felt familiar. I was a woman in a workplace where men held the positions of power and I was being overlooked, not heard. But, then, in that same breath, there you were. With your boisterous voice echoing up to the ceiling and back down, you interrupted the director's thought and corrected his false assumption. Never one to hesitate to give credit where it's due, you also challenged the gender bias at play.

The exchange was brief, but it has lived on inside me ever since. It's in the knowledge that, although I am strong-willed and fully capable of standing up for myself, at times I might falter. You were there for me, backing me up, showing the heart, humility, and kindness it takes to stand up for someone else. I thank you.

Your #1 fan,

—*Jessica Stroup*, LOS ANGELES, CALIFORNIA

do >

Give recognition to someone who rarely receives it.

Life starts out with lots of encouragement, but the amount of praise we get from others tends to sharply fall off as we age. There is an expectation to toil quietly, endlessly, and thanklessly. Defy expectations. Be a cheerleader for someone who has none.

learn >

Self-compassion has been linked to traits such as **cognitive wisdom**, curiosity, personal initiative, **happiness**, and optimism.

(NEFF ET AL. 2007)

reflect >

KINDER.

Honestly, I can be so mean to myself.

My own worst critic.

The world's laziest judge who doesn't take the time to
look at the facts

But decides to find everything wrong

And make it a song of negative opinions whose lyrics

Lock me up in a cell of headspace clouded with negativity.

The walls are engraved with the words "you're worthless." It's lonely.

The cold drafts freeze me in time, convincing me to fear that this will
last forever.

And I tell myself that everything is wrong about me and I'm wrong
about everything . . . except for that.

It will last forever.

When I finally escape, the world goes from black and white to color

And I realize I could have been kinder.

Instead of reading the words "I'm worthless," I should've said, "I'm worth it."

I should have recognized the warmth inside my heart.

I now see that nothing about me is wrong. Nothing about you is wrong.

We're human.

Science shows us that kindness can improve your mental health. And kindness includes kindness to self. Securing our own oxygen masks first will smoothen out the move for us to be kinder to each other.

So be a little kinder to my friend for me, and yes, my friend, is you.

— *Malick Mercier,* BROOKLYN, NEW YORK

do >

Forgive yourself for a past social faux pas.

Have you been meaning to return your grandma's phone call, thank a friend for going out of their way for you, or answer an email that has been been sitting in your inbox for months? Well, it's never too late to acknowledge you received that call, help, or email! Forgiving yourself for first not responding will enable you to cut through the awkwardness and reestablish that social connection.

learn >

Kindness is beautiful.

People who are generous receive higher attractiveness ratings than those who are not.

(ARNOCKY ET AL. 2017)

week 46

199

reflect >

Q & A WITH TOM TAIT

Tom Tait is the former mayor of Anaheim, California (2010 to 2018).

You went from being a lawyer, to working in a family business, to being on the city council in Anaheim, California. What a journey!

Nothing happened as I imagined. I always had a terrible fear of speaking and then wound up in law. Then, through a series of bizarre circumstances, I was appointed to serve on the city council. I was there until I reached limit terms in 2004. And for six years, I saw so many broken moments in our community. We're a city of 350,000 people, and I felt frustrated that we were treating the symptoms over and over again with the same solutions, but treating those symptoms wasn't nearly enough.

And then you ran for mayor—and did so on a platform of kindness?

Yes, crazy sounding, I know. But when the mayor seat opened up in 2010, I felt that I needed to run. And my fears of public speaking were still real. I was scared of being ridiculed. But I had a conviction—something deep within that I had to try—even if I lost. I had seen these signs around town saying "kindness is contagious," and the word was like a hidden gem to me. What would our community be like if we are a city of kindness? The entire campaign I said I wanted to lead with kindness, be a mayor who helped make kindness a core value of our city, and I ended up being elected.

Did it work? Did you see a difference?

Well, I was reelected for a second term! What I learned is that it is truly all the small acts of kindness that create meaningful impact and develop a city culture. From initiatives focused on getting to know your neighbors better, to building community resiliency, to cleaning up our streets and recycling more, to reducing bullying in schools—all of those things we work on in cities—everything gets better by developing a culture of kindness.

do >

Learn how to recycle something you didn't know you could.

Recycling glass bottles and plastics #1, #2, and #3 are all well and good, but you can do more. Many communities offer programs beyond garbage collection. Among the materials they accept are batteries, certain kinds of light bulbs, appliances, used cooking oil, and packing materials, like bubble wrap and gel freeze packs. The planet can use all the kindness it can get.

learn >

Expressing **gratitude improves the well-being** of both expressers and recipients (and expressers undervalue its positive impact on recipients).

(KUMAR AND EPLEY 2018)

week 47

203

reflect >

HAVE I EVER THANKED YOU?

Dear Mary,

I can't describe how much you have meant, and still mean, to me. I'm so deeply grateful for your friendship. In the more than twenty years we have known each other, you have done so much to help me. Just being there to listen to me, you were the first one who really showed me the power of active listening. I learn so much from you every time we get together. I can't think of anyone who has been so kind and selfless in giving and caring.

And yet, I realize that I've never taken the time to tell you how deeply you've impacted my life until now. As I look back, I can remember so many wonderful things you've done for me. I don't know why I've never expressed how grateful I am for our relationship, that the universe connected us, and that you, probably more than anyone else in my life, have always been there for me.

Thank you for everything, Mary. From the depths of my heart and soul, thank you.

—*Jack Abbott*

"For me, my daily act of kindness is to open my heart and lend an ear to anyone who needs it—to help someone feel that what they have to say matters."

—DIANE HOUSLIN

do >

Write someone a letter—a real letter, on paper—and mail it!

There's something so personal about putting pen to paper, and the fact that it's increasingly rare to receive anything handwritten makes it even more special. Use a fun stamp or colorful envelope, get playful with your greeting, doodle a picture—anything to make it stand out from the usual junk mail and bills. It's such a simple way to brighten someone's day.

learn >

Someone needs blood **every 2 seconds** in the United States. 1 pint of blood can **save up to 3 lives**.

(AMERICAN RED CROSS 2019)

reflect >

TAKING THE FEAR OUT
OF GIVING BLOOD

I had never donated blood, but my wife is a cancer survivor and blood saved her life. So, one year, I thought, *I'll try this*. I'm now a regular donor, and my blood type, AB negative, is the rarest kind (less than 0.5 percent of the population has it, making the need for donors that much more important). Every time I walk into a donor center, the thank-yous and smiles are unbelievable. It costs me nothing, and yet, what I am giving is priceless. It can save lives.

Before I knew the power of donating blood, I used to think it would be a burden to do it, to have to sit in a chair for twenty to thirty minutes, experience the needles, see the blood. But once I did it, I wanted to keep doing it. I know how much every time matters.

But the really beautiful part of it all is how my four-year-old son reacts to it. The first time, he thought I would die. Now, I try to bring him with me every single time, because I want him to know that donating blood is normal, not something to be scared of. The questions he throws at me can make it fun: Daddy, where is all this blood going? Why? But I hope he will grow up thinking of this as normal behavior and become a donor himself.

—*Basil Hatto,* **TORONTO, CANADA**

do >

Donate blood.

Parting with the very fluid your body needs to survive sounds intense, especially if you're not a fan of needles. But consider how amazing it is that every human body is designed to give a portion of its lifesaving force to another. Perhaps nature itself is driven to be kind. Giving blood could very well be the easiest opportunity to save a life. Find a location convenient to you and make an appointment. Blood banks are rarely fully stocked, so the need is constant.

learn >

week 49

"Compassion is a program made of neural tissue. The program is triggered when it **detects that someone is in need**. When activated, the program coordinates our attention and thoughts. So, if we value a person's welfare or if they are in great need, we act on the compassionate impulse and help."

—*Daniel Sznycer,* ASSISTANT PROFESSOR OF PSYCHOLOGY AT THE UNIVERSITY OF MONTREAL

211

reflect >

Q & A WITH HENRY HITCHCOX

Henry Hitchcox is a multi-award-winning filmmaker and creative director.

You've created multiple films and campaigns about kindness that have received hundreds of millions of views. What have these productions taught you, and have they changed the way you go about your day-to-day life?

When I first began shooting stunts and documentaries about kindness, my focus (and that of the cameras!) was naturally on the person receiving the kind act. However, I quickly started to notice the more subtle and often profound reaction of the giver. No matter how big or small the act, it was always clear that they were deriving real pleasure from being kind. We needed to capture that too—kindness is just as beautiful and joyous for the giver as it is for the receiver.

"Be kind, for everyone you meet is fighting a hard battle."

—JOHN WATSON

do >

Plant postcards of positivity.

Grab a card or sticky note and write something encouraging ("You'll get through this!"), happy ("It's a beautiful day!"), or funny ("You smell great!") and leave it in the work break room, at a bus stop, or in a random bathroom stall. Words have weight, and yours could tip the balance of someone's day from bad to good when they least expect it.

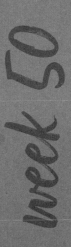

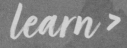learn >

People who spent time **helping others** felt that **they had more time** themselves.

(MOGILNER ET AL. 2012)

reflect >

COLLECTIVE KINDNESS SAVES THE DAY

Soon after I moved to New York City, I was riding a crowded F train. Like many, the subway is not my favorite place in the world. I tend to zone out to make the ride more bearable, but I noticed the woman next to me frantically looking around. I asked if she was okay, and she explained she had lost an earring. I helped her look but came up empty-handed. I asked the person next to me if they could look too.

Before I knew it, the message had been passed around and everyone in the subway car was looking. Sure enough, the person at the very end of the car found her gold hoop. The earrings had been passed down from her grandmother, so they were very special to her. And—just like that—everyone went back to doing their own thing. But I think we all felt a little more energized as we went about our day.

That moment taught me a lot about New York. Yes, there's lots of hustle, but there's also an underlying current of togetherness and community.

—*Amelia Erikson,* NEW YORK, NEW YORK

"No act of kindness,
no matter how small,
is ever wasted."

—AESOP

do >

Volunteer your time.

Volunteering doesn't have to wait until your schedule clears up. With time, like with money, just give what you can. Maybe you can't commit to being a volunteer firefighter, but you can sign up to walk dogs at your local shelter once a month, take part in a community cleanup day, or give a few minutes when someone needs help with something. Whatever you can do, it helps.

learn >

Acts of kindness and generosity **trigger** activity in **happiness**-related areas of the brain [such as the ventral striatum].

(PARK ET AL. 2017)

reflect >

Q & A WITH ERIC RIPERT

Eric Ripert is a French chef, author, and television personality.

Professional kitchens are often perceived as abusive settings. Many chefs think it is necessary, and par for the course in a top-rated kitchen. How did you break out of that thinking?

I was an angry chef, too, at first. It was all I knew. It was how I was trained, and I knew it was expected from me. I would have no problem taking plates and throwing them on the floor. I didn't have the space for happiness. It took years to break from that tradition. I started to meditate. At first it was very difficult and tedious. Today, it is a real pleasure to be able to meditate. In the kitchen, we are firm in our orders because you need to have a certain authority, but I don't see our cooks scared or shaking. Without screaming, without intimidating, I call it "the kind approach."

"Kindness, I've discovered, is everything in life."

—ISAAC BASHEVIS SINGER

do >

Share a meal with someone who usually eats alone.

We bond over food like few other things, and it plays such a central role in family celebrations that having no one to break bread with can feel especially isolating. If a neighbor, colleague, or friend is dining alone, it may not be by choice, but due to the loss of a loved one (to death or divorce), a recent move to the area, or other circumstance. A family dinner, even if it isn't with their family, can be a welcome change.

learn >

Kindness is **millions of years old**. It originally evolved to motivate care of offspring; later, the psychology was co-opted to support cooperative relationships **beyond the family**.

(CURRY ET AL. 2018)

reflect >

DEAR YOU

Dear You (reading this now),

I've spent a great deal of my life empowering women to choose kindness and compassion, both for themselves and others. And I want to humbly share my personal experience, which time and time again, I am reminded of the simple fact that kindness feels better in my body. I find that the weight of resentment, anger, bitterness, and cynicism are simply too heavy, too demanding, and too exhausting to carry.

There is a warmth about kindness—my chest relaxes, I breathe deeper, my shoulders fall—and I'm no longer bound by angst, stress, or irritation. My words slow down, along with my heartbeat, and I sink into a comfortable, almost imperceptible lull that makes smiling easier and laughing more accessible.

So, my advice is this, choose kindness in a world where it can feel like it's unseen. Choose it for no other reason than that it simply feels better inside your body, because it's sugar to your soul, sweet balm to your emotions, and a sanctuary for your mind to rest. Love you more. Love you most. Choose kindness.

Always,

—*Lex*

"That's the power
of kindness, it can
rewrite the ending."

—KINDNESS.ORG

do >

What's your kindness story?

Congratulations on completing 52 weeks of kind acts! Do you feel different? Sharing kindness is spreading kindness, and we'd love to know the impact this book has had on you. Has your definition of kindness changed? What was the most impactful act you did or received? We want to hear anything you have to share with us. **Submit your story at kindness.org/bekind or email us at bekind@kindness.org.**

Notes

Notes

Notes

Kind Acts Checklist

○ Identify kindness in the wild.

○ Send a thank-you text. Unprovoked.

○ Connect with a co-worker.

○ Consider how to combine honesty and compassion.

○ Book a date with yourself.

○ Be mindful of opportunities to help as they arise.

○ Pay a stranger's way.

○ Count your blessings. Literally.

○ Ask if you can help with anything.

○ Spend some time in nature.

○ Forgive a past wrong.

○ Stand, so someone else can sit.

○ Reconnect with someone you haven't seen in a while.

○ Give an occasion-free gift to a loved one or co-worker.

○ Let someone go ahead of you in a long line.

○ Acknowledge someone when they walk into the room.

○ Respond kindly to a negative comment online.

○ Encourage a friend who's struggling.

○ Donate to a worthy cause.

○ Invite someone to join you in completing a kind act.

○ Take a nap.

○ Set a daily gratitude reminder on your phone.

○ Give a book away.

○ Learn how to become an organ donor.

- ⭕ Thank someone who made a difference in your life.
- ⭕ Try a smile experiment.
- ⭕ Spend quality time with an elderly person.
- ⭕ Turn your no into a yes.
- ⭕ Play! Do something fun.
- ⭕ Treat someone without even being there.
- ⭕ Apologize from the heart.
- ⭕ Take time to get informed.
- ⭕ Get to know your neighbors.
- ⭕ Clean up someone else's act.
- ⭕ Share your knowledge with someone.
- ⭕ Learn the name of a person you see regularly.
- ⭕ Give future you a boost.
- ⭕ Earmark a five-dollar bill for random acts of kindness.
- ⭕ Give meditation a go.
- ⭕ Choose kindness, even in the face of its opposite.
- ⭕ Talk to a child about kindness.
- ⭕ Change your bad mood with a good deed.
- ⭕ Give recognition to someone who rarely receives it.
- ⭕ Forgive yourself for a past social faux pas.
- ⭕ Learn how to recycle something you didn't know you could.
- ⭕ Write someone a letter on paper and mail it.
- ⭕ Donate blood.
- ⭕ Plant postcards of positivity.
- ⭕ Volunteer your time.
- ⭕ Share a meal with someone who usually eats alone.
- ⭕ Share your kindness story.

Bibliography

Aknin, Lara B., Alice L. Fleerackers, and J. Kiley Hamlin. "Can Third-Party Observers Detect the Emotional Rewards of Generous Spending?" *Journal of Positive Psychology* 9, no. 3 (2014): 198–203.

American Red Cross. "Blood Needs & Blood Supply." American Red Cross online, 2019, https://www.redcrossblood.org/donate-blood/how-to-donate/how-blood-donations-help/blood-needs-blood-supply.html.

Anderson, G. Oscar, and Colette Thayer. "Loneliness and Social Connections: A National Survey of Adults 45 and Older." AARP online, September 2018, https://www.aarp.org/research/topics/life/info-2018/loneliness-social-connections.html.

Arnocky, Steven, Tina Piché, Graham Albert, Danielle Ouellette, and Pat Barclay. "Altruism Predicts Mating Success in Humans." *British Journal of Psychology* 108, no. 2 (2017): 416–35.

Breines, Julian G., and Serena Chen. "Self-Compassion Increases Self-Improvement Motivation." *Personality and Social Psychology Bulletin* 38, no. 9 (2012): 1133–43.

Cassandra. Cassandra Report: The Impact Issue. Cassandra online, 2016, https://cassandra.co/reports/2016/03/24/impact.

Chancellor, Joseph, Seth Margolis, Katherine Jacobs Bao, and Sonja Lyubomirsky. "Everyday Prosociality in the Workplace: The Reinforcing Benefits of Giving, Getting, and Glimpsing." *Emotion* 18, no. 4 (2018): 507–17.

Curry, Oliver Scott, Lee A. Rowland, Caspar J. Van Lissa, Sally Zlotowitz, John McAlaney, and Harvey Whitehouse. "Happy to Help? A Systematic Review and Meta-Analysis of the Effects of Performing Acts of Kindness on the Well-Being of the Actor." *Journal of Experimental Social Psychology* 76 (2018): 320–29.

Dickens, Leah R. "Using Gratitude to Promote Positive Change: A Series of Meta-Analyses Investigating the Effectiveness of Gratitude Interventions." *Basic and Applied Social Psychology* 39, no. 4 (2017): 193–208.

Dunn, Elizabeth W., Lara B. Aknin, and Michael I. Norton. "Spending Money on Others Promotes Happiness." *Science* 319, no. 5870 (2008): 1687–88.

Fowler, James H., and Nicholas A. Christakis. "Cooperative Behavior Cascades in Human Social Networks." *PNAS* 107, no. 12 (2010): 5334–38.

Hardy, Charlie L., and Mark Van Vugt. "Nice Guys Finish First: The Competitive Altruism Hypothesis." *Personality and Social Psychology Bulletin* 32, no. 10 (2006): 1402–13.

Khoury, Bassam, Manoj Sharma, Sarah E. Rush, and Claude Fournier. "Mindfulness-Based Stress Reduction for Healthy Individuals: A Meta-Analysis." *Journal of Psychosomatic Research,* 78, no. 6 (2015): 519–28.

Kraft-Todd, Gordon T., and David G. Rand. "Rare and Costly Prosocial Behaviors Are Perceived as Heroic." *Frontiers in Psychology* 10 (2019): 234.

Kumar, Amit, and Nicholas Epley. "Undervaluing Gratitude: Expressers Misunderstand the Consequences of Showing Appreciation." *Psychological Science* 29, no. 9 (2018): 1423–35.

Leary, Mark R., Eleanor B. Tate, Claire E. Adams, Ashley Batts Allen, and Jessica Hancock. "Self-Compassion and Reactions to Unpleasant Self-Relevant Events: The Implications of Treating Oneself Kindly." *Journal of Personality and Social Psychology* 92, no. 5 (2007): 887–904.

Lundahl, Brad W., Mary Jane Taylor, Ryan Stevenson, and K. Daniel Roberts. "Process-Based Forgiveness Interventions: A Meta-Analytic Review." *Research on Social Work Practice* 18, no. 5 (2008): 465–78.

McCullough, Michael E., Lindsey M. Root, and Adam D. Cohen. "Writing about the Benefits of an Interpersonal Transgression Facilitates Forgiveness." *Journal of Consulting and Clinical Psychology* 74, no. 5 (2006): 887–97.

McGrath, Robert E. "Character Strengths in 75 Nations: An Update." *The Journal of Positive Psychology* 10 no. 1 (2014): 41–52.

Mogilner, Cassie, Zoë Chance, and Michael I. Norton. "Giving Time Gives You Time." *Psychological Science* 23, no. 10 (2012): 1233–38.

Neely, Michelle E., Diane L. Schallert, Sarojanni S. Mohammed, Rochelle M. Roberts, and Yu-Jung Chen. "Self-Kindness When Facing Stress: The Role of Self-Compassion, Goal Regulation, and Support in College Students' Well-Being." *Motivation and Emotion* 33, no. 1 (2009): 88–97.

Neff, Kristin D., Stephanie S. Rude, and Kristin L. Kirkpatrick. "An Examination of Self-Compassion in Relation to Positive Psychological Functioning and Personality Traits." *Journal of Research in Personality* 41, no. 4 (2007): 908–16.

Park, Soyoung Q., Thorsten Kahnt, Azade Dogan, Sabrina Strang, Ernst Fehr, and Philippe N. Tobler. "A Neural Link between Generosity and Happiness." *Nature Communications* 8 (2017): 15964.

Parker, Laura. "Ocean Trash: 5.25 Trillion Pieces and Counting, but Big Questions Remain. *National Geographic* online, January 11, 2015, https://www.nationalgeographic.com/news/2015/1/150109-oceans-plastic-sea-trash-science-marine-debris/.

Petelczyc, Claire Aislinn, Alessandra Capezio, Lu Wang, Simon Lloyd D. Restubog, and Karl Aquino. "Play at Work: An Integrative Review and Agenda for Future Research." *Journal of Management* 44, no. 1 (2018): 161–90.

Pew Research Center. "Teaching the Children: Sharp Ideological Differences, Some Common Ground." Pew Research Center online, September 18, 2014, https://www.people-press.org/2014/09/18/teaching-the-children-sharp-ideological-differences-some-common-ground.

Pressman, Sarah D., Tara L. Kraft, and Marie P. Cross. "It's Good to Do Good and Receive Good: The Impact of a 'Pay It Forward' Style Kindness Intervention on Giver and Receiver Well-Being." *The Journal of Positive Psychology* 10, no. 4 (2015): 293–302.

Raposa, Elizabeth B., Holly B. Laws, and Emily B. Ansell. "Prosocial Behavior Mitigates the Negative Effects of Stress in Everyday Life." *Clinical Psychological Science: A Journal of the Association for Psychological Science* 4, no. 4 (2016): 691–98.

Roberts, Hannah, Caspar van Lissa, Paulien Hagedoorn, Ian Kellar, and Marco Helbich. "The Effect of Short-Term Exposure to the Natural Environment on Depressive Mood: A Systematic Review and Meta-Analysis." *Environmental Research* 177 (2019): 108606.

Rosekind, Mark R., R. Curtis Graeber, David F. Dinges, Linda J. Connell, Michael S. Rountree, Cheryl L. Spinweber, and Kelly A. Gillen. "Crew Factors in Flight Operations 9: Effects of Planned Cockpit Rest on Crew Performance and Alertness in Long-Haul Operations." NASA online, September 1, 1994, https://ntrs.nasa.gov/search.jsp?R=19950006379.

Steger, Michael F., Brian M. Hicks, Todd B. Kashdan, Robert F. Krueger, and Thomas J. Bouchard Jr. "Genetic and Environmental Influences on the Positive Traits of the Values in Action Classification, and Biometric Covariance with Normal Personality." *Journal of Research in Personality* 41, no. 3 (2007): 524–39.

Thomas, Ashley J., Lotte Thomsen, Angela F. Lukowski, Meline Abramyan, and Barbara W. Sarnecka. "Toddlers Prefer Those Who Win but Not When They Win by Force." *Nature Human Behaviour* 2, no. 9 (2018): 662–69.

Trew, Jennifer L., and Lynn E. Alden. "Kindness Reduces Avoidance Goals in Socially Anxious Individuals." *Motivation and Emotion* 39, no. 6 (2015): 892–907.

U.S. Chamber of Commerce Foundation. "Business of Kindness." U.S. Chamber of Commerce Foundation online, 2017, https://www.uschamberfoundation.org/business-kindness.

Van Oudenhoven, Jan Pieter, Boele de Raad, Marieke E. Timmerman, François Askevis-Leherpeux, Pawel Boski, Carmen Carmona, Rajneesh Choubisa, Alejandra del Carmen Dominguez, Hege H. Bye, Anastacia Kurylo, Cornelia Lahmann, Khairul Mastor, Eva Selenko, Alena Slezáčková. Ripley Smith, Linda Tip, and Michelle Yik. "Are Virtues National, Supranational, or Universal?" *Springerplus* 3 (2014): 223.

Whillans, Ashley V., Elizabeth W. Dunn, G. M. Sandstrom, Sally S. Dickerson, and K. M. Madden. "Is Spending Money on Others Good for Your Heart?" *Health Psychology* 35, no. 6 (2016): 574–83.

Acknowledgments

We've long said this mission is only made possible by the people around the world who put it into action every day. This book is no exception. There are so many people who helped make it possible and we're incredibly grateful for each one of you.

To Rage, Erin, Laura, Cara, Lydia, and the entire Quarto publishing team, thank you for caring deeply about creating a book like this. We are grateful for your time, your passion, and can't wait to see what more we do together.

Thank you to Neil, our third co-founder, who, through your support and heart and desire for a kinder world, we've been able to dream big and build something to help make kindness the norm. Thinking makes it so.

Writing a book while also running an organization takes an incredible support system. Thank you to Oliver, Genevieve, Marlon, Gabe, Taylor, Sydni, Eva, and Thalia, for being all hands on deck to research, organize, react, and celebrate at all the right times. Paula, thank you for the gift of your time and for truly seeing us. Jill, thank you for jumping in at a moment's notice and for your words of encouragement. Sarah, thank you for putting words to this work. Amelia, thank you for building a kindness community.

Thank you to our board of directors, Mike, Yukari, Aditya, and Sergio, for supporting us so well during this season.

Thank you to our wonderful community members across 192 nations—people who have signed on to champion kindness where they live, work, and go to school. To each and every person who has joined us in building a kinder world, we thank you.

And last but definitely not least, thank you to our wonderful families for being patient, for reading multiple drafts, for helping with mealtimes and bedtimes for our kids, and for continuing to be our biggest champions. We couldn't have done this without you.

About the Authors

MELISSA BURMESTER, co-founder and chief product officer of kindness.org, loves asking questions and building teams to solve complex problems. She is an author, keynote speaker, and start-up advisor. Throughout her career, she has produced content from eight different countries, conducted countless interviews, and amassed over 160 million video views. Working closely with kindness.org's research team to study the impact of kindness, Melissa helps leverage their findings to create new programs that can be implemented in schools and workplaces. She avidly believes that kindness transcends difference. Outside of work, Melissa is passionate about volunteering at organizations focused on disaster relief, education, and ending childhood hunger. You can catch her hosting living-room dance parties with her young daughter every Saturday morning.

JACLYN LINDSEY, co-founder and CEO of kindness.org, believes that kindness is humanity's greatest asset. It was this ethos that inspired her to launch kindness.org, a global non-profit building evidence-based programs for kinder classrooms, communities, and workplaces. Jaclyn has spent over a decade in the nonprofit space, where she has helped raise more than $100 million for domestic and international missions. An author and keynote speaker, she sits on the board of Children in Conflict and is an advisor to Creative Mint and Expectful. When not whiteboarding ways to use kindness for good, Jaclyn loves adventuring around with her husband, Mancel, and son, Abel, and spending time with family, friends, or strangers around a dinner table.

About Kindness.org

Kindness.org is a research-led nonprofit dedicated to educating and inspiring people to choose kindness. Through their research hub, Kindlab, they investigate the costs and benefits of kindness, and the role it can play in solving modern problems. With the help of more than four hundred volunteer citizen scientists and a global community representing 192 nations, they test academic findings in the real world. They then take their learnings and create products and programs to bring kindness to classrooms, communities, and workplaces around the world. Learn Kind, an inquiry-based learning framework for bringing kindness and social-emotional education to classrooms, was recently launched for this purpose. Work Kind serves a similar purpose for businesses, using action-based programming to maximize the well-being of organizations and the people who power them. All these efforts contribute to the vision of a world where kindness is at the forefront of human interaction.